a LANGE medical book

CURRENT
Practice Guidelines
In Primary Care
2005

D1081243

Ralph Gonzales, MD, MSPH

Associate Professor
Division of General Internal Medicine
Department of Medicine
University of California, San Francisco
San Francisco, California

Jean S. Kutner, MD, MSPH

Associate Professor and Interim Chief
Division of General Internal Medicine
Department of Medicine
University of Colorado Health Sciences Center
Denver, Colorado

Lange Medical Books/McGraw-Hill
Medical Publishing Division

New York   Chicago   San Francisco   Lisbon   London
Madrid   Mexico City   Milan   New Delhi   San Juan   Seoul
Singapore   Sydney   Toronto

The McGraw-Hill Companies

CURRENT Practice Guidelines in Primary Care, 2005

1 2 3 4 5 6 7 8 9 0 DOC/DOC 0 9 8 7 6 5 4

ISBN: 0-07-145098-X
ISSN: 1528-1612

Notice

Medicine is an ever-changing science. As new research and clinical experience broaden our knowledge, changes in treatment and drug therapy are required. The authors and the publisher of this work have checked with sources believed to be reliable in their efforts to provide information that is complete and generally in accord with the standards accepted at the time of publication. However, in view of the possibility of human error or changes in medical sciences, neither the authors nor the publisher nor any other party who has been involved in the preparation or publication of this work warrants that the information contained herein is in every respect accurate or complete, and they disclaim all responsibility for any errors or omissions or for the results obtained from use of the information contained in this work. Readers are encouraged to confirm the information contained herein with other sources. For example and in particular, readers are advised to check the product information sheet included in the package of each drug they plan to administer to be certain that the information contained in this work is accurate and that changes have not been made in the recommended dose or in the contraindications for administration. This recommendation is of particular importance in connection with new or infrequently used drugs.

This book was set in Times New Roman by Silverchair Science + Communications.
The editor was Janet Foltin.
The production supervisor was Phil Galea.
RR Donnelley was the printer and binder.
This book is printed on acid-free paper.

Contents

1. DISEASE SCREENING

"√" denotes major 2005 updates.
* denotes important new evidence since latest guideline(s) published.

2. DISEASE PREVENTION

"√" denotes major 2005 updates.
* denotes important new evidence since latest guideline(s) published.

3. DISEASE MANAGEMENT

"√ " denotes major 2005 updates.
* denotes important new evidence since latest guideline(s) published.

4. APPENDICES

"√ " denotes major 2005 updates.
* denotes important new evidence since latest guideline(s) published.

"√ " denotes major 2005 updates.
* denotes important new evidence since latest guideline(s) published.

Preface

Current Practice Guidelines in Primary Care, 2005 is intended for primary care clinicians. These include not only residents and practicing physicians in the specialties of family medicine, internal medicine, pediatrics, and obstetrics and gynecology but also medical and nursing students during their ambulatory care rotations, registered nurses, nurse practitioners, and physician assistants. Its purpose is to make *screening, primary prevention*, and *management* recommendations readily accessible and available for clinical decision making. The recommendations included are issued regularly by governmental agencies, expert panels, medical specialty organizations, and other professional and scientific organizations.

Current Practice Guidelines in Primary Care, 2005 is essential for the busy clinician. New recommendations are continually being published by organizations that express different positions on the same topics, and current guidelines require revision as new evidence from clinical and outcomes research emerges. The intent of this guide is both to help clinicians select the most appropriate clinical preventive services and interventions for a given situation and to provide clinicians with quick access to the latest information.

Current Practice Guidelines in Primary Care, 2005 has been updated using PubMed searches limited to articles published in English between 10/20/03 and 7/24/04 and "practice guideline" publication type, as well as via the websites of major professional societies, the Agency for Healthcare Research and Quality Guidelines Clearinghouse, and the U.S. Preventive Services Task Force. This updating strategy led to substantial modification of many guidelines (look for "√" in the Contents). New material has been added addressing management of metabolic syndrome, palliative and end-of-life care issues, prenatal care, and smoking cessation. We are grateful to Dr. Jennifer Adams for her careful reviews and editing assistance.

Ralph Gonzales, MD, MSPH
Associate Professor
University of California, San Francisco
San Francisco, California

Jean S. Kutner, MD, MSPH
Associate Professor and Interim Chief
University of Colorado Health Sciences Center
Denver, Colorado

December 2004

1
Disease Screening

ALCOHOL ABUSE & DEPENDENCE

Disease Screening	Organization	Date	Population	Recommendations	Comments	Source
Alcohol Abuse & Dependence	AAP BrightFutures GAPS	2001 1997 1997	Adolescents	Ask all adolescents annually about their use of alcohol.	1. Parents should routinely receive instructions on monitoring their adolescent's social and recreational activities for use of alcohol.[a] 2. The finding of alcohol use or abuse should provoke an assessment of other conditions that co-vary with alcohol abuse, such as cigarette smoking, sexual activity, and mood disorders.	Arch Pediatr Adolesc Med 1997;151:123 Pediatrics 1995;95:439
	AMA USPSTF ASAM	2004 2004 1997	Adults	Screen all adults using relevant history or a standardized screening instrument. Implement brief behavioral counseling interventions to reduce alcohol misuse.[c]	3. Guidelines on treatment of alcohol abuse in adolescence have been published. (J Am Acad Child Adolesc Psychiatry 1998;37:122) 4. A systematic review concluded that the Alcohol Use Disorders Identification Test (AUDIT) was most effective in identifying subjects with at-risk, hazardous, or harmful drinking (sensitivity, 51%–79%; specificity, 78%–96%); while the CAGE questions proved superior for detecting alcohol abuse and dependence (sensitivity, 43%–94%; specificity 70%–97%). (Arch Intern Med 2000;160:1977)[b]	Ann Intern Med 2004;14():7)
	NIAAA	2002	College students	Screen all students on National Alcohol Screening Day.[d]	5. Screening coupled with brief physician advice is cost-effective (Med Care 2000;38:7) and produces small to moderate reductions in alcohol consumption. 6. Light to moderate alcohol consumption has been associated with some health benefits in nonpregnant adults, including reduced risk for coronary artery disease.	http://www.collegedrinkingprevention.gov

ALCOHOL ABUSE & DEPENDENCE

Disease Screening	Organization	Date	Population	Recommendations	Comments	Source
Alcohol Abuse & Dependence (continued)					7. 1,400 college students between the ages of 18 and 24 die each year from alcohol-related injuries. (J Studies Alcohol 2002;63:136) 8. Targeting only those with identified problems misses students who drink heavily or misuse alcohol occasionally. Nondependent, high-risk drinkers account for majority of alcohol-related deaths and damage.	
	AAP ACOG	1997	Pregnant women	Counsel all pregnant women regarding the maternal health and fetal effects of alcohol during pregnancy.		AAP and ACOG: Guidelines for Perinatal Care, 4th ed. ACOG, 1997

[a]The AAP also acknowledges the importance of family attitudes toward alcohol and recommends that clinicians urge parents to use alcohol safely and in moderation, to restrict children from family alcohol supplies, and to recognize the influence their own drinking patterns can have on their children and parenting.
[b]See Appendix I: Screening Instruments, Alcohol Abuse for CAGE and AUDIT instruments.
[c]Hazardous drinking is defined as more than 7 drinks per week for women and more than 14 drinks per week for men. Harmful drinking describes people with physical, social, or psychological harm from drinking who do not meet criteria for dependence. (Arch Intern Med 1999;159)
[d]National Alcohol Screening Day is April 7, 2005; sponsored by the National Institute on Alcohol Abuse and Alcoholism and other organizations (http://mentalhealthscreening.org/alcohol.asp).

Disease Screening	Organization	Date	Population	Recommendations	Comments	Source
ANEMIA						
Anemia	AAP	1993	Neonates	Universal hematocrit screening is not recommended.		Pediatrics 1993;92:474
	AAFP USPSTF	2002 1996	Infants aged 6–12 months	Perform selective, single hemoglobin or hematocrit screening for high-risk infants.[a]		
	CDC	1998	Infants and preschool children at high risk (migrants, refugees, and low income)	Screen high-risk children for anemia between 9 and 12 months, 6 months later, and annually from 2 to 5 years.		MMWR 1998;47:RR-3
			Adolescent and adult women	Screen all nonpregnant women beginning in adolescence every 5–10 years until menopause.	1. When acute stress or inflammatory disorders are not present, a serum ferritin level is the most accurate test for evaluating iron deficiency anemia.	
	CDC USPSTF	1998 1996	Pregnant women	Screen all women with hemoglobin or hematocrit at first prenatal visit.	Among women of childbearing age, a cut-off of 15 mg/dL has sensitivity of 75%, specificity of 98%. (Br J Haematol 1993;85:787)	

[a]Includes infants living in poverty, blacks, Native Americans and Alaska Natives, immigrants from developing countries, preterm and low birthweight infants, and infants whose principal dietary intake is unfortified cow's milk.

CANCER, BLADDER

Disease Screening	Organization	Date	Population	Recommendations	Comments	Source
Cancer, Bladder	AAFP USPSTF CTF	2004 2004 1994	Asymptomatic persons	Routine screening with microscopic urinalysis, urine dipstick, or urine cytology is *not* recommended.	1. Dipstick testing is sensitive and specific for hematuria, but hematuria is not specific for bladder cancer. 2. A high index of suspicion should be maintained in anyone with a history of smoking or exposure to another risk factor.[a]	http://www.aafp.org/exam.xml
	NCI	2004	Asymptomatic persons	There is insufficient evidence to determine whether a decrease in mortality occurs with screening of any type.	3. People who smoke should be advised that smoking significantly increases the risk for bladder cancer, and all smokers should be routinely counseled to quit smoking (OR/RR 1.5–7.0). 4. Other tests, such as bladder tumor antigen, NMP22 urinary enzyme immunoassay, and urine cytology, are of unproven benefit in screening for bladder cancer.	http://www.cancer.gov/cancer_information/testing

[a]Increased risk: exposure to azodyes, aromatic amines, and 4-aminobiphenyl; employment in the leather, tire, or rubber industries; neuropathic bladder; chronic indwelling catheter; and cigarette smoking. Persons working in high-risk professions may be eligible for screening at the worksite, although the benefit of this has not been determined.

Disease Screening	Organization	Date	Population	Recommendations[a,b]	Comments	Source
Cancer, Breast	ACS CTF	2004 2001	Women aged ≥ 20 years	Women should be told about the benefits and limitations of BSE. It is acceptable for women to choose not to do BSE or to do it occasionally.	1. The value of BSE in reducing breast cancer mortality remains unproved. (Br J Cancer 1993;68:208) 2. The CBE should be conducted close in time to the scheduled mammogram. A normal mammogram in the presence of a palpable mass does not rule out breast cancer.	http://www.cancer.org http://www.ctfphc.org
	ASCO	2003	Women aged ≥ 20 years	Monthly BSE. Recommend against screening for genetic mutations in the general population.[d]	3. It is likely that < 10% of all breast cancer in Western countries is attributable to genetic predisposition, but 25% of breast cancers diagnosed before age 40 years are attributable to *BRCA1* mutations.[c] These women may benefit from more frequent mammography as well as earlier initiation of mammogram and/or the addition of breast ultrasound or MRI. (ACS) 4. 30% of all women screened annually at ages 40–49 will have at least 1 false-positive mammogram. (J Natl Cancer Inst 1997;22:139)	http://www.asco.org
	ACS AMA ASCO ACOG	2004 2004 2003 2002	Women aged 20–39 years	CBE every 3 years.		http://www.cancer.org http://www.ama-assn.org http://www.asco.org http://www.acog.org
	AAFP NCI	2004 2004	Women aged ≥ 40 years	Mammography every 1–2 years.	5. Extending screening to include ages 40–49 improves life expectancy by 2.5 years at a cost of $676 per woman. Incremental cost-effectiveness is $105,000 per year of life saved. (Ann Intern Med 1997;127:955)	http://www.aafp.org/exam.xml http://cancernet.nci.nih.gov http://www.cancer.gov/cancertopics/types/breast

CANCER, BREAST

Disease Screening	Organization	Date	Population	Recommendations[a, b]	Comments	Source
Cancer, Breast (continued)	ACS AMA ASCO ACOG ACR	2004 2004 2003 2002 2002	Women aged ≥ 40 years	Mammography and CBE yearly.	6. RCTs consistently demonstrate no benefit from screening in the first 5–7 years after study entry. At 10–12 years, benefit is uncertain. [J Natl Cancer Inst 1993;85(20):1644] 7. Number needed to screen to save 1 life = 2,500. [J Natl Cancer Inst 1997;89(14):1015] 8. Risk-based recommendations may assist in counseling. [J Clin Oncol 1998;16(9):3105]	http://www.cancer.org http://www.ama-assn.org http://www.asco.org http://www.acog.org http://www.acr.org CA Cancer J Clin 2002;52.8–22
	USPSTF	2002	Women aged ≥ 40 years	Mammography, with or without CBE, every 1–2 years.	9. Screening women aged 50–69 years improves life expectancy by 12 years at a cost of $704 per woman, with a cost-effectiveness ratio of $21,400 per year of life saved. (Ann Intern Med 1997;127:955)	http://www.ahrq.gov/clinic/3rduspstf/breastcancer
	CTF	2001	Women aged 40–49 years	Counsel about risks/benefits of mammography and CBE.	10. Present data are insufficient to recommend use of tumor markers (CA15-3, CEA) for screening for breast cancer.	CMAJ 2001;164(4):469–476 http://www.ctfphc.org
	AMA ACP	2004 1991	Women aged 50–69 years	Mammography and CBE yearly.		http://www.ama-assn.org http://www.acponline.org JAMA 1989;261(17):2535
	CTF ACPM	1998 1996	Women aged 50–69 years	Mammography and CBE every 1–2 years.		http://www.ctfphc.org http://www.acpm.org/breast.htm

CANCER, BREAST					

Disease Screening	Organization	Date	Population	Recommendations[a, b]	Comments	Source
Cancer, Breast (continued)	AGS ACPM	1999 1996	Women aged ≥ 70 years	Mammography and CBE every 1–2 years, with no upper age limit for women with an estimated life expectancy of ≥4 years. AGS recommends, in addition, monthly BSE.	1. Currently available data for women aged > 70 are inadequate to judge the effectiveness of screening. [J Natl Cancer Inst 1993;85(20):1644] 2. Screening mammography in frail older women frequently necessitates work-up that offers no benefit. Encouraging individualized decisions may allow screening to be targeted to older women for whom the potential benefit outweighs the potential burdens. (J Gen Intern Med 2001;16:779–784) 3. Extending biennial screening to age 75–80 is estimated to cost $34,000–$88,000 per life-year gained. It is most cost-effective to target healthy women rather than those with several competing risks for death. [Ann Intern Med 2003;139(10)]	http://www.american geriatrics.org http://www.acpm.org/breast.htm

[a]Debate about the value of screening mammograms was triggered by a Cochrane review published on October 20, 2001. (Lancet 2001;358:1340–1342) This review cited a number of methodologic and analytic flaws in the large long-term mammography trials. The USPSTF and NCI concluded that the flaws were problematic but unlikely to negate the consistent and significant mortality reductions observed in the trials.

[b]Summary of current evidence: NEJM 2003;348:1672–1680.

[c]In one study, nearly half of BRCA-positive women developed malignant disease detected by mammography less than 1 year after a normal screening mammogram. [Cancer 2004;100(10)]

[d]Women who present with early-onset disease (< 50 years), multiple or bilateral tumors, or family history may benefit from genetic testing. (ASCO) Referral to a specialized center for comprehensive genetic counseling services is appropriate.

CANCER, CERVICAL

Disease Screening	Organization	Date	Population	Recommendations	Comments	Source
Cancer, Cervical	ACOG ACS	2004 2004	Women within 3 years after first sexual intercourse or by age 21, whichever comes first[a]	Annual Pap smear until age 30 (every 2 years if liquid-based Pap test, ACS).[b] At age ≥ 30, if 3 consecutive normal results, may screen every 2–3 years. Continue to screen annually if risk factors present. If negative on *both* Pap smear and HPV DNA test, rescreen with combined tests every 3 years.[c]	1. Cervical cancer is causally related to infection with HPV. (http://odp.od.nih.gov/) 2. Other risk factors include early onset of sexual intercourse; history of multiple sexual partners or male sexual partners who have had multiple partners; male partners whose other sexual partners have had cervical cancer; history of STDs (especially HPV, HIV, HSV); immunosuppression; smoking; history of cervical dysplasia or endometrial, vaginal, or vulvar cancer; and no previous screening. 3. Long-term use of oral contraceptives may increase risk of cervical cancer in women who are positive for cervical human papillomavirus DNA. (Lancet 2002;359:1085) 4. 20%–60% reduction in cervical cancer mortality rates after implementation of screening programs. [Ann Intern Med 1990;113(3):214] Most cases of cervical cancer occur in women who are not screened adequately. (USPSTF) 5. Lead time from precancerous lesions to invasive cancer is 8–9 years. (Clinician's Handbook of Preventive Services. U.S. Government Printing Office, 1994) 6. Single screening Pap test for detecting CIN grades I and II has sensitivity 14%–99%, specificity 24%–96%. (Am J Epidemiol 1995;141:680)	http://www.acog.org http://www.cancer.org Ann Intern Med 2000;133:1021–1024 Ann Intern Med 1990;113(3):214
	ASCO	2003	Women within 3 years after first sexual intercourse or by age 21, whichever comes first[a]	Pap smear at least every 2–3 years.		http://www.asco.org
	Bright Futures GAPS	2002 1994	Women who are or have been sexually active[a]	Pap smear and pelvic exam every year; if > 3 consecutive normal exams, may perform less frequently at physician discretion.[c]		http://www.brightfutures.org

Disease Screening	Organization	Date	Population	Recommendations	Comments	Source
Cancer, Cervical (continued)	NCI	2002	Women who are or have been sexually active **OR** Women aged > 18 years[a]	Regular screening with Pap smear decreases mortality. The upper age limit at which screening ceases to be effective is unknown.	7. The rate of false-negative results from HPV DNA testing may be as high as 50%. An estimated 1/2 to 2/3 of false-negative results are caused by inadequate specimen collection and by misinterpreting or not observing abnormal cells. HPV DNA testing may have a strong role in identifying precancerous lesions and managing minor Pap abnormalities. (Ann Intern Med 2000;133:1021–1024) 8. Preliminary evidence suggests that a vaccine against HPV-16 significantly reduces the risk of acquiring transient and persistent infection and cervical cancer. (NEJM 2002;347)	http://cancernet. nci.nih.gov
	USPSTF AAFP ACP	2003 2002 1990	Women who have ever had sex and have a cervix[a]	Pap smear at least every 3 years.[d]		http://www.aafp. org/exam.xml Ann Intern Med 1990;113(3):214
	ACOG ACS ASCO USPSTF	2004 2004 2003 2003	Women without a cervix	Discontinue routine Pap smear screening in women who have had a total hysterectomy for benign disease and no history of abnormal cell growth.		

CANCER, CERVICAL

CANCER, CERVICAL						
Disease Screening	Organization	Date	Population	Recommendations	Comments	Source
Cancer, Cervical (continued)	ACPM CTF	1996 1994	Women who have ever had sex[a]	Pap smear every year for 2 years; if 2 normal annual smears, lengthen screening interval to 3 years at physician discretion.[c]		http://www.acpm. org/cervical.htm
	ACS ASCO USPSTF ACPM	2004 2003 2003 1996	Women aged > 65 years (aged > 70 years, ACS)	Discontinue screening if: at least 2 normal smears within previous 10 years, and not otherwise at high risk for cervical cancer. If no previous screening, 3 normal smears before discontinuation.	1. 28%–64% of women aged > 65 have never had a Pap smear or have not had one done within 3 years. (Mt Sinai J Med 1985;52:284) 2. In one study, women 65 years of age and older were 21% less likely than younger women to ever have had a Pap test and 33% less likely to have had a Pap test recently. Physician recommendation is the strongest predictor of whether a woman receives a Pap test. (Ann Intern Med 2000;133:1021–1024) 3. Beyond age 70, there is little evidence for or against screening women who have been regularly screened in previous years. Individual circumstances such as the patient's life expectancy, ability to undergo treatment if cancer is detected, and ability to cooperate with and tolerate the Pap smear procedure may obviate the need for cervical cancer screening.	http://www.asco. org http://www.cancer. org http://www.acpm. org/cervical.htm
	AGS CTF	2000 1994	Women aged > 65 years	Pap smear every 1–3 years until age 70. If no or insufficient prior Pap smears, 2 annual smears before discontinuation.		http://www.ameri cangeriatrics.org/ products/position papers/cer_care_ 2000.shtml J Am Geriatr Soc 2001;49:655

[a]If sexual history is unknown or considered unreliable, screening should begin at age 18 years.
[b]New tests to improve cancer detection include liquid-based/thin-layer preparations, computer-assisted screening methods, and human papillomavirus testing. (Am Fam Phys 2001;64:729)
[c]As compared with annual screening for 3 years, screening performed once every 3 years after the last negative test in women aged 30–64 years who have had ≥ 3 consecutive negative Pap smears is associated with an average excess risk of approximately 3 in 100,000. (NEJM 2003;349:1501–1509)
[d]USPSTF notes that most of the benefit can be obtained by beginning screening within 3 years of onset of sexual activity or age 21.

CANCER, COLORECTAL

Disease Screening	Organization	Date	Population	Recommendations	Comments	Source
Cancer, Colorectal	ACS ACG ACP AGA ASGE USPSTF	2004 2003 2003 2003 2003 2002	Aged ≥ 50 years at average risk[a]	Screen with 1 of the following strategies:[b, c, d] 1) FOBT annually[e] 2) Flexible sigmoidoscopy every 5 years 3) FOBT annually plus flexible sigmoidoscopy every 5 years 4) Colonoscopy every 10 years 5) Double-contrast barium enema every 5 years	1. A positive screening test should be followed by colonoscopy.[f] 2. Approximately half of patients with proximal neoplasms had no distal lesions. Therefore, yearly FOBT and flexible sigmoidoscopy is preferred to either alone. (ACS) However, in a prospective study, one-time screening with FOBT and sigmoidoscopy fails to detect 24% of subjects with advanced colonic neoplasia. (NEJM 2001;345:555) 3. Patients should be involved in a shared decision-making process for choosing the most appropriate screening test. The choice should be based on patient preferences, medical contraindications, patient adherence, and resources for testing and follow-up. (USPSTF) 4. Models indicate that screening persons > 50 years for colorectal cancer with annual FOBT, flexible sigmoidoscopy, or a single colonoscopy compares favorably with screening mammography in women aged > 50 years in the cost per year of life saved. [NEJM 1995;332(13):861]	Gastroenterology 2003;124;544 NEJM 2000;343:162 NEJM 2000;343:169 CA Cancer J Clin 2001;51:38 http://caonline.amcancersoc.org/cgi/content/full/51/1/3 http://www.ahrq.gov/clinic/uspstf/uspscolo.htm Ann Intern Med 2002;137:129 http://cancernet.nci.nih.gov/
	AAFP	2004	Aged ≥ 50 years[a]	"Recommends, not strongly" Yearly FOBT,[b,c] flexible sigmoidoscopy, colonoscopy, or barium enema		http://www.aafp.org/exam.xml
	ASCRS	1999	Aged ≥ 50 years, low or average risk[a]	Yearly DRE and 1 of the following: FOBT[b,c] and flexible sigmoidoscopy every 5 years OR Total colon exam (colonoscopy or double-contrast barium enema and proctosigmoidoscopy)		http://www.fascrs.org/

Disease Screening	Organization	Date	Population	Recommendations	Comments	Source
Cancer, Colorectal (continued)	ACS ACG ACP AGA ASGE	2004 2003 2003 2003 2003	Persons at increased risk based on family history[g]	*Group I:* Screening colonoscopy at age 40 years, or 10 years younger than the earliest diagnosis in their family, and repeated every 5 years. *Group II:* Follow average risk recommendations, but begin at age 40 years. *Group III:* see Average Risk	5. Screening for colorectal cancer, even in the setting of imperfect compliance, significantly reduces colorectal cancer mortality at costs comparable to other cancer screening procedures. (JAMA 2000;284:1954–1961) 6. FOBT alone decreased colorectal cancer mortality by 33% compared with those who were not screened. (Gastroenterology 2004;126) 7. New techniques such as CT virtual colonoscopy are not recommended as screening at this time.	

[a]Risk factors indicating need for earlier/more frequent screening: personal history of colorectal cancer or adenomatous polyps, colorectal cancer or polyps in a first-degree relative < 60 years old or in a second-degree relative of any age, personal history of chronic inflammatory bowel disease, and family with hereditary colorectal cancer syndromes. [Ann Intern Med 1998;128(1):900, NEJM 1994;331(25):1669, NEJM 1995;332(13):861] If history of colorectal cancer in first-degree relative, age 55 years or younger, or 2 or more first-degree relatives of any ages, colonoscopy is recommended at age 40 or 10 years before the youngest case in the family, whichever is earlier. (http://www.fascrs.org)

[b]A positive result on an FOBT should be followed by colonoscopy. An alternative is flexible sigmoidoscopy and air-contrast BE.

[c]FOBT should be performed on 2 samples from 3 consecutive specimens obtained at home.

[d]USPSTF did not find direct evidence that screening colonoscopy is effective in reducing colorectal cancer mortality rates.

[e]Use the guaiac-based test with dietary restriction, or an immunochemical test without dietary restriction. Two samples from each of 3 consecutive stools should be examined without rehydration. Rehydration increases the false-positive rate.

[f]Colonoscopy is the preferred test. If not available, double-contrast barium enema and flexible sigmoidoscopy should be performed.

[g]*Group I:* First-degree relative with colon cancer or adenomatous polyps at age ≤ 60 years, or 2 first-degree relatives with colorectal cancer at any time. *Group II:* First-degree relative with colon cancer or adenomatous polyp at age ≤ 60 years, or 2 first-degree relatives with colorectal cancer. *Group III:* 1 second-degree or third-degree relative with colorectal cancer.

DRE = digital rectal exam; FOBT = fecal occult blood testing

Disease Screening	Organization	Date	Population	Recommendations	Comments	Source
Cancer, Endometrial	ACS	2004	All women	Routine screening of women for endometrial cancer is not recommended.	1. Presence of endometrial cells in Pap test from postmenopausal women not taking exogenous hormones is abnormal and requires further evaluation. Pap test is insensitive for endometrial screening.	CA Cancer J Clin 2001;51:54
	NCI	2002	All women	There is insufficient evidence that screening with endometrial sampling or transvaginal ultrasound decreases mortality.	2. Endometrial thickness of < 4 mm on transvaginal ultrasound is associated with low risk of endometrial cancer. [Obstet Gynecol 1991;78(2):195]	http://cancernet.nci.nih.gov/
	AAFP ACS	2004 2004	All women at high risk for endometrial cancer.[a]	Annual screening at age 35 years with endometrial biopsy.	1. Variable screening with ultrasound among women (aged 25–65 years; $n = 292$) at high risk for HNPCC mutation detected no cancers from ultrasound. Two endometrial cases occurred in the cohort that presented with symptoms. (Cancer 2002;94:1708) 2. One should also consider that the RR of endometrial cancer associated with tamoxifen use in women with breast cancer is approximately 1.5 overall, and increases to RR = 6.9 for women taking tamoxifen for at least 5 years. (Lancet 2000;356:881) 3. The WHI demonstrated that combined estrogen and progestin did not increase risk of endometrial cancer but did increase rate of endometrial biopsies and ultrasound exams prompted by abnormal uterine bleeding. (JAMA 2003;290)	CA Cancer J Clin 2001;51:54

[a]High-risk women are those known to carry hereditary nonpolyposis colorectal cancer–associated genetic mutations, or at high risk to carry mutation, or who are from families with suspected autosomal dominant predisposition to colon cancer.
HNPCC = hereditary nonpolyposis colorectal cancer; WHI = Womens' Health Initiative

CANCER, GASTRIC					
Disease Screening	Organization	Date	Population	Recommendations	Comments	Source
Cancer, Gastric	NCI	2004	Adults in the United States	There is insufficient evidence to establish that screening would result in a decrease in mortality from gastric cancer in the U.S. population.	1. Perhaps due to the higher incidence of gastric cancer in Japan, studies of screening in Japan (via barium x-ray) have demonstrated decreases in mortality in screened vs. unscreened patients. (Int.J Cancer 1995;60:45)	http://cancernet.nci.nih.gov/

	CANCER, LIVER					
Disease Screening	Organization	Date	Population	Recommendations	Comments	Source
Cancer, Liver (Hepatocellular Carcinoma, HCC)	NCI	2004	Children and adults	There is insufficient evidence to establish that screening by alpha fetoprotein (AFP) and/or imaging techniques (eg, CT or ultrasound) would result in a decrease in mortality from HCC.	1. Chronic hepatitis B and C are the major risk factors for HCC. In the United States, chronic hepatitis B and C account for ~30%–40% of HCC. Other risk factors: alcoholic cirrhosis, hemochromatosis, alpha-1-antitrypsin deficiency, glycogen storage disease, porphyria cutanea tarda, tyrosinemia, Wilson's disease. 20%–50% of patients presenting with HCC have previously undiagnosed cirrhosis.	http://www.cancernet.nci.nih.gov
	British Society of Gastroenterology	2003	Adults	Surveillance with abdominal ultrasound and AFP every 6 months should be considered for high-risk groups.[a]	2. Patients should be made aware of the implications of early diagnosis and lack of proven survival benefit. 3. Patients with single small HCC (≤5 cm) or up to 3 lesions ≤ 3 cm should be referred for assessment for hepatic resection or transplantation.	Gut 2003;52(Suppl III):iii

[a]All persons with established cirrhosis with HBV, HCV, or hemachromatosis; males with cirrhosis due to alcohol or primary biliary cirrhosis.

	CANCER, LUNG				
Disease Screening	Organization	Date	Population	Recommendations	Comments	Source

Disease Screening	Organization	Date	Population	Recommendations	Comments	Source
Cancer, Lung	AAFP NCI ACCP ACS CTF	2004 2004 2003 2002 1994	Asymptomatic persons	Routine screening for lung cancer with CXR, sputum cytology, or low-dose CT (LDCT) is not recommended.	1. Counsel all patients against tobacco use. Over 50 years, men who continued to smoke died, on average, 10 years earlier than lifelong nonsmokers. Smokers who quit gain life expectancy. (BMJ 2004;328) 2. No significant benefit in terms of lung cancer mortality by screening with CXR and sputum cytology. (J Occup Med 1986;28:746) 3. Annual low-dose chest CT in high-risk patients appears to increase detection of resectable cancer. Impact of screening on mortality has not been determined. (Lancet 1999;354:99–105) There should be no compromise or shortcuts in the rigorous scientific process required to determine whether lung cancer screening is justified. (http://www.uicc.org, NEJM 2000;343:1627, JAMA 2000;284:1980) 4. The NCI is conducting the National Lung Screening Test (NLST), an RCT comparing LDCT and CXR for detecting and reducing lung cancer mortality among persons at risk for lung cancer. (http://www.cancer.org)	http://cancernet.nci.nih.gov http://www.aafp.org/exam.xml http://www.cancer.org The Medical Letter 2001;43(1109):61–62 Chest 2003;123:835–885
	USPSTF	2004	Asymptomatic persons	Evidence is insufficient to recommend for or against lung cancer screening.		

Disease Screening	Organization	Date	Population	Recommendations	Comments	Source
CANCER, ORAL						
Cancer, Oral	NCI USPSTF CTF	2004 2004 1999	Asymptomatic persons	Smoking cessation counseling (CTF). There is insufficient evidence to establish that screening would result in a decrease in mortality from oral cancer.	1. Risk factors: regular alcohol or tobacco use.	http://cancernet.nci.nih.gov/ J Can Dent Assoc 1999;65:617
	NIDR	1994	Asymptomatic persons	Screen during routine dental exam.		Detecting Oral Cancer: A Guide for Dentists. NIDR, 1994.
	CTF	1999	High-risk persons[a]	Consider annual oral exam.		

[a]Inquire about alcohol and tobacco use and counsel about risk.

Disease Screening	Organization	Date	Population	Recommendations	Comments	Source
Cancer, Ovarian	AAFP NCI USPSTF ASCO ACPM	2004 2004 2004 2003 1997	Asymptomatic women[a]	There is insufficient evidence to establish that screening for ovarian cancer with serum markers such as CA-125 levels, transvaginal ultrasound, or pelvic examinations would result in a decrease in mortality from ovarian cancer.[b]	1. Risk factors: aged > 60 years; low parity; personal history of endometrial, colon, or breast cancer; family history of ovarian cancer; and hereditary ovarian cancer syndrome. Use of oral contraceptives decreases risk of ovarian cancer. 2. In asymptomatic women, pelvic exam has unknown sensitivity and specificity; abdominal ultrasound has specificity 97.7%, sensitivity 100%, positive predictive value 2.6%; transvaginal ultrasound has specificity 98.1%, sensitivity 100%, positive predictive value 22%; CA-125 has sensitivity 50% for stages I and II and 90% for stages III and IV, and specificity 97.6%, when followed by abdominal ultrasound. [Ann Intern Med 1993;118(11):838; http://www.acpm.org/ovary.htm] 3. There are no data demonstrating that screening high-risk women reduces their mortality from ovarian cancer.[c]	http://www.aafp.org/exam.xml http://www.asco.org http://www.cancernet.nci.nih.gov/ http://www.acpm.org/ovary.htm
	ACOG ASCO ACS	2003 2003 2002	Asymptomatic women[a]	Recommend physical examination every 3 years in women aged 20–39 years, and annually in women aged ≥ 40 years.		http://www.acog.org http://www.asco.org CA Cancer J Clin 2002;52:8
	NIH	1994	Asymptomatic women[a]	Comprehensive family history and annual rectovaginal pelvic exam		NIH Consensus Statement 1994;12(3):1

[a] Lifetime risk of ovarian cancer in a woman with no affected relatives is 1 in 70. If 1 first-degree relative has ovarian cancer, lifetime risk is 5%. If 2 or more first-degree relatives have ovarian cancer, lifetime risk is 7%. Women with 2 or more family members affected by ovarian cancer have a 3% chance of having a hereditary ovarian cancer syndrome. These women have a 40% lifetime risk of ovarian cancer.

[b] Several large-scale studies designed to establish the effectiveness of general population screening for ovarian cancer have begun. Each uses transvaginal ultrasonography or a multimodal strategy in which elevated serum levels of CA-125 tumor marker prompt secondary testing with transvaginal ultrasonography. (Ann Intern Med 2000;133:1021–1024)

[c] A low annual incidence (13.8/100,000) means that many people must be screened to find only a few cases of disease. [NIH Consensus Statement 1994;12(3):1, Ann Intern Med 1993;118(11):838]

CANCER, OVARIAN

CANCER, PANCREATIC

Disease Screening	Organization	Date	Population	Recommendations	Comments	Source
Cancer, Pancreatic	AAFP USPSTF CTF	2004 2004 1994	Asymptomatic persons	Routine screening using abdominal palpation, ultrasonography, or serologic markers is not recommended.	1. Cigarette smoking has consistently been associated with increased risk of pancreatic cancer.	http://www.aafp.org/exam.xml

CANCER, PROSTATE						

Disease Screening	Organization	Date	Population	Recommendations	Comments	Source
Cancer, Prostate	NCI	2004	Asymptomatic men	Insufficient evidence to establish whether a decrease in mortality from prostate cancer occurs with screening by DRE or serum PSA.	1. There is good evidence that PSA can detect early-stage prostate cancer, but mixed and inconclusive evidence that early detection improves health outcomes or mortality. 2. DRE has sensitivity 50%, specificity 94%; PSA has sensitivity 67%, specificity 84%; TRUS has sensitivity 81%, specificity 84%. [JAMA 1994;272(10):773]	http://cancernet.nci.nih.gov/
	AAFP USPSTF	2004 2002	Asymptomatic men Aged 50–65 years (AAFP)	Evidence insufficient to recommend for or against routine screening using PSA or DRE.	3. Further evaluation is recommended when PSA > 4. However, a recent study found an overall prevalence of prostate cancer of 15% in men with a PSA < 4. (NEJM 2004:350) Because we do not	http://www.aafp.org/exam.xml
	ACS AUA	2004 2003	Men aged ≥ 50 years[a]	Offer annual PSA and DRE if > 10-year life expectancy.[b]	know which tumors are clinically significant, lowering the threshold for biopsy at this time is not recommended. 4. Screening with PSA or DRE detects some cancers that would not have been clinically significant, leading to overtreatment. Treatments including prostatectomy and radiation can result in permanent erectile dysfunction and urinary incontinence (NCI).	http://www.cancer.org Oncology 2000;14:267–286 http://auanet.org

				CANCER, PROSTATE	
Disease Screening	Organization	Date	Population	Recommendations	Comments	Source
Cancer, Prostate (continued)	ACPM ACP	1998 1997	Men aged > 50 years[a]	Describe potential benefits and known harms of screening with PSA and DRE, diagnosis, and treatment; listen to the patient's concerns; and individualize the decision to screen.	1. PSA rise of > 2 per year is associated with recurrence and death. (NEJM 2004;351) It is not known if using PSA velocity to determine treatment is useful. 2. A recent RCT using finasteride for chemoprevention of prostate cancer showed a reduced incidence of cancer in the treatment group but a greater proportion of high-grade tumors. Therefore, this strategy is not recommended. (NEJM 2003;349)	http://www.acpm. org/prostate.htm Ann Intern Med 1997;126(6):480

[a]Men in high-risk groups (2 or more affected first-degree relatives, blacks) should begin screening at age 40. If PSA < 1.0 ng/mL, no additional testing is needed until age 45. If PSA 1.0–2.5 ng/mL, annual testing is recommended. If PSA ≥ 2.5 ng/mL, consider further evaluation with biopsy. More data on the precise age to start prostate cancer screening are needed for men at high risk. No direct or indirect evidence quantifies the yield and predictive value of early detection efforts in higher-risk men. [http://www.cancer.org/, http://auanet.org/, Ann Intern Med 1997;126(6):480]

[b]Some elevations in PSA may be due to benign conditions of the prostate. The DRE should be performed by health care workers skilled in recognizing subtle prostate abnormalities, including those of symmetry and consistency, as well as the more classic findings of marked induration or nodules. DRE is less effective in detecting prostate carcinoma than is PSA. (http://www.cancer.org/, http://auanet.org/)

Disease Screening	Organization	Date	Population	Recommendations	Comments	Source
CANCER, SKIN						
Cancer, Skin	AAFP NCI USPSTF	2004 2004 2003	Asymptomatic persons	Insufficient evidence to recommend for or against routine screening using total-body skin exam.[a, b] **OR** Counseling patients to perform periodic skin self-exam.[c]	1. Appropriate biopsy specimens should be taken of suspicious lesions. Persons with melanocytic precursor or marker lesions are at substantially increased risk for malignant melanoma and should be referred to skin cancer specialists for evaluation and surveillance. (USPSTF)	http://cancernet.nci.nih.gov/ http://www.aafp.org/exam.xml
	ACPM	1998	Asymptomatic persons	Periodic total cutaneous examinations, targeting populations at high risk for malignant melanoma.[c] Insufficient evidence to characterize periodicity of skin examinations more precisely.		http://www.acpm.org/skincanc.htm
	ACS	2004	Aged 20–39 years	Screening with physician skin exam every 3 years. Self-exam every month.		http://www.cancer.org
	ACS	2004	Aged ≥ 40 years	Annual screening with physician skin exam. Self-exam every month.		http://www.cancer.org

[a]Clinicians should remain alert for skin lesions with malignant features when examining patients for other reasons, particularly patients with established risk factors. Risk factors for skin cancer include: evidence of melanocytic precursors, large numbers of common moles, immunosuppression, family or personal history of skin cancer, substantial cumulative lifetime sun exposure, intermittent intense sun exposure or severe sunburns in childhood, freckles, poor tanning ability, and light skin, hair, and eye color.

[b]NCI notes that, based on poor evidence, visual examination of the skin leads to a reduction in mortality from melanoma skin cancer.

[c]Consider educating patients with established risk factors for skin cancer (see above) concerning signs and symptoms suggesting skin cancer and the possible benefits of periodic self-exam. (USPSTF)

Disease Screening	Organization	Date	Population	Recommendations	Comments	Source
CANCER, TESTICULAR						
Cancer, Testicular	NCI CTF	2004 1994	Asymptomatic men	Insufficient evidence to recommend for or against routine screening by physician exam, patient self-exam, or tumor markers (alpha fetoprotein, human chorionic gonadotropin)	1. Insufficient evidence to establish that screening would result in a decrease in mortality from testicular cancer, in part because treatment at each stage is very effective, the prevalence is very low, and screening tests are of limited accuracy.	http://cancernet.nci.nih.gov/
	USPSTF	2004	Asymptomatic men[a]	Recommend against screening asymptomatic men		

[a] Patients with history of cryptorchidism, orchiopexy, or testicular atrophy should be informed of their increased risk for developing testicular cancer and counseled about screening. Such patients may then elect to be screened or to perform testicular self-exam. Adolescent and young adult males should be advised to seek prompt medical attention if they notice a scrotal abnormality. (USPSTF)

	CANCER, THYROID				

Disease Screening	Organization	Date	Population	Recommendations	Comments	Source
Cancer, Thyroid	AAFP USPSTF CTF	2004 1996 1994	Asymptomatic persons	Screening asymptomatic adults or children using either neck palpation or ultrasonography is not recommended.[a]	1. Neck palpation for nodules in asymptomatic individuals has sensitivity 15%–38%; specificity 93%–100%. Only a small proportion of nodular thyroid glands are neoplastic, resulting in a high false-positive rate. (USPSTF)	http://www.aafp.org/exam.xml

[a]Includes asymptomatic persons with a history of external upper-body irradiation in infancy or childhood.

Disease Screening	Organization	Date	Population	Recommendations	Comments	Source
Carotid Artery Stenosis (asymptomatic)						**CAROTID ARTERY STENOSIS**
	AHA	1998	Aged 40–79 years	Screen asymptomatic patients (? interval) with < 5% surgical risk and > 5-year life expectancy.[a]	1. In the Asymptomatic Carotid Atherosclerosis Study (ACAS), the actuarial 5-year risk of ipsilateral stroke, operative stroke, and death was ≅ 5% with CEA vs. 11% in the control group. Combined surgical morbidity and mortality was 2.3%. (JAMA 1995;273:1421) In ACAS, the benefit of surgery was greater for men than women (reduction in risk 66% vs. 17%).	http://circ.ahajournals.org/cgi/content/full/97/5/501
	CNS	1997	Aged 40–79 years	Insufficient evidence to screen asymptomatic individuals because recommendation is "uncertain" for > 60% stenosis.[b]	2. The cumulative cost-effectiveness of targeted screening and surgery for high-grade carotid artery stenosis is ~$43,000 per QALY. (MJM 1999;5:35–41) 3. The prevalence of internal carotid artery stenosis (ICAS) of ≥ 70% is low in persons with only atherosclerosis risk factors (1.8%–2.3%), intermediate in those with angina or MI (3.1%), and highest in those with PAD (12.5%) or AAA (8.8%). Advanced age (> 54	Can Med Assoc J 1997;157:653
	USPSTF	1996	Aged > 60 years	Selective screening.[c]	years) and lower diastolic BP (< 83 mm Hg) increased prevalence of ICAS. (J Vasc Surg 2003;37:1226–1233) 4. The Asymptomatic Carotid Surgery Trial (ACST) is the largest trial to date. (Lancet 2004;363:1491) The absolute risk reduction for stroke or death at 5 years was 5.4%, with significant benefit observed in women (4% absolute risk reduction) as well as in men (8.2% risk reduction).	

CAROTID ARTERY STENOSIS

[a]If surgical risk is < 3% and life expectancy is > 5 years, ipsilateral CEA is acceptable for > 60% stenosis; if surgical risk is 3–5%, ipsilateral CEA is acceptable (but not proved) for > 75% bilateral stenoses.

[b]Recommend stenosis be documented with angiography using the method of the North American Symptomatic Carotid Endarterectomy Trial.

[c]Selective screening may be appropriate in the presence of other stroke risk factors, no contraindications to major surgery, and access to surgeons and centers with < 3% perioperative morbidity and mortality.

CHILD ABUSE & NEGLECT

Disease Screening	Organization	Date	Population	Recommendations	Comments	Source
Child Abuse & Neglect	USPSTF	2004	Children	Insufficient evidence to recommend for or against routine screening.	1. By law, child abuse must be reported to appropriate authorities in all 50 states.	Ann Fam Med 2004;2:156–160
	AAFP AAP ACOG Family Violence Prevention Fund NAPNAP	2002	Children and adolescents	Screen caregivers/parents and adolescents at new patient visits, at least once per year, and when new intimate relationship. Ask when signs and symptoms raise concerns (physical signs, behavioral or emotional problems, chronic somatic complications).		http://www.endabuse.org
	GAPS	1997	Children and adolescents	All teens should be asked annually about a history of emotional, physical, and sexual abuse.		Arch Pediatr Adolesc Med 1997;151:123

CHLAMYDIAL INFECTION

Disease Screening	Organization	Date	Population	Recommendations	Comments	Source
Chlamydial Infection	ACPM	2003	Sexually active women	Annually screen high-risk women.[a]	1. Antigen detection tests and nonamplified nucleic acid hybridization, as well as newer amplified DNA assays, may provide improved sensitivity, lower expense, availability, and/or timeliness of results over culture. 2. Noninvasive methods such as urine specimens and vaginal swabs appear reliable. 3. Early detection and treatment of women at risk for chlamydial infection (prevalence 7%) reduced the incidence of pelvic inflammatory disease from 28 per 1,000 woman-years to 13 per 1,000 woman-years. Ecologic studies also show a decrease in ectopic pregnancy with the advent of community-based chlamydial screening programs. 4. Recent population-based studies show overall prevalence of chlamydial infection in 18–26-year-old persons to be 4.7%, with rates sixfold higher among African Americans. Most surprisingly, prevalence rates in men were 3.5%. (JAMA 2004;291:2229)	Am J Prev Med 2003;24:287
	AAFP	2004	Women aged ≤25 years who are sexually active	Strongly recommends screening.		
	USPSTF	2001	Women aged ≤25 years who are sexually active or pregnant	Routinely screen for chlamydial infection; the optimal interval for screening is uncertain.[b]		
	ACPM	2003	Pregnant women	Screen during their first trimester or first prenatal visit.		Am J Prev Med 2003;24:287

[a]Aged ≤25 years, new male sex partners or 2 or more partners during preceding year, inconsistent use of barrier methods, history of prior STD, African-American race, cervical ectopy.
[b]For women with a previous negative screening test, the interval for rescreening should take into account changes in sexual partners. If there is evidence that a woman is at low risk for infection (eg, in a mutually monogamous relationship with a previous history of negative screening tests for chlamydial infection), it may not be necessary to screen frequently. Rescreening at 6 to 12 months may be appropriate for previously infected women because of high rates of reinfection.

CHOLESTEROL & LIPID DISORDERS, CHILDREN

Disease Screening	Organization	Date	Population	Recommendations	Comments	Source
Cholesterol & Lipid Disorders, Children	AACE AAP	2000 1998	Aged > 2 years	Selective screening[a] every 5 years if normal[b] Fasting lipids if strong family history Random total cholesterol if a parent has total cholesterol ≥ 240 mg/dL Clinician discretion (random total cholesterol) if unknown family history or presence of risk factors	1. Recommend pharmacologic treatment (eg, cholestyramine or colestipol) if: (1) age > 10 years, on dietary therapy, and LDL ≥ 190 mg/dL without other risk factors; or (2) LDL ≥ 160 mg/dL and strong family history or 2 or more risk factors are present.[a] See management algorithms.	Endocr Pract 2000 Mar–Apr;6:162–213 Pediatrics 1998;101:141–147
	USPSTF	1996	Children and adolescents	Insufficient evidence to recommend for or against screening		

CHOLESTEROL & LIPID DISORDERS, ADULTS

Disease Screening	Organization	Date	Population	Recommendations	Comments	Source
Cholesterol & Lipid Disorders, Adults	NCEP III AACE	2002 2000	Men and women aged > 20 years	Check fasting lipoprotein panel (if testing opportunity is non-fasting, use TC and HDL) every 5 years if in desirable range; otherwise see management algorithm.[b]	1. NCEP III modifies recommendations (vs. NCEP II) to promote more aggressive primary prevention (ie, intensive lipid lowering) in persons with multiple risk factors for CHD. 2. Optimal interval for screening is uncertain. 3. Age to stop screening is not established. Clinical trial data demonstrate that persons older than 65 years of age derive the same benefit from cholesterol reduction as younger adults. 4. Base treatment decisions on at least 2 cholesterol levels.	Circulation 2002;106:3143 http://www.nhlbi.nih.gov/guidelines/cholesterol/atp3upd04.htm Endocr Pract 2000 Mar–Apr;6:162–213
	USPSTF AAFP	2001	Men aged 20–35 years Women aged 20–45 years	Selective screening of individuals with major CHD risk factors [hypertension, smoking, diabetes, family history of CHD before age 50 (male relatives) or age 60 (female relatives), family history suggestive of familial hyperlipidemia]		
	AAFP USPSTF	2002 2001	Men aged ≥ 35 years Women aged ≥ 45 years	"Strongly recommended" Random total cholesterol and HDL cholesterol or fasting lipid profile, periodicity based on risk factors		Am J Prev Med 2001;20(35):73–76 http://www.aafp.org/exam.xml Geriatrics 2003;58:33–38

[a]AAP recommends annual screening if strong family history (parents or grandparents) of cardiovascular events at or before age 55 years (MI, positive coronary angiogram, stroke, peripheral vascular disease, or sudden cardiac death) or presence of "several" risk factors (cigarette smoking, hypertension, obesity, diabetes, lack of physical activity).
[b]Classify TC < 200 mg/dL as desirable, 200–239 mg/dL as borderline, or ≥ 240 mg/dL as high. Classify HDL < 40 as low, and ≥ 60 as high. Classify LDL < 100 as optimal, 100–129 as near or above optimal, 130–159 as borderline high, 160–189 as high, and ≥ 190 as very high. If TC < 200 mg/dL and HDL ≥ 40 mg/dL, then repeat in 5 years; if TC ≥ 200 mg/dL or HDL < 40 mg/dL, then check fasting lipids and risk stratify based on LDL (see management algorithm).

| | | | | | DEMENTIA | |

Disease Screening	Organization	Date	Population	Recommendations	Comments	Source
Dementia	AHCPR	1996	Elderly	Perform selective screening[a] using a standardized instrument to assess cognitive function.[b]	1. Screening instruments are useful for detecting multiple cognitive deficits and determining a baseline for future assessments. 2. Reversible causes of dementia include vitamin B_{12} deficiency, neurosyphilis, and hypothyroidism. Be aware of other causes of mental status changes, such as depression, delirium, medication effects, and coexisting illnesses. 3. The additional benefit of identifying early dementia is to prepare family for future patient needs. 4. Clock Drawing Test is a valid screening method for cognitive impairment. (Dement Geriatr Cogn Disord 2004;18:172–179)	J Am Geriatr Soc 1988;37:562 Activities of daily living: J Am Geriatr Soc 1985;33:698 Mini Mental Status Exam: J Psychiatr Res 1975;12:189, also see Mini Mental State Examination in Appendix 1
	USPSTF AAN CTF	2003 2001 2001	Elderly, asymptomatic	Insufficient evidence to recommend for or against routine screening for dementia.		Ann Intern Med 2003;138:925–926 Ann Intern Med 2003;138:927–937 Neurology 2001;56:1133–1142
	AGS AAN	2003 2001	Elderly, Mild Cognitive Impairment (MCI)[d]	Persons with MCI should be evaluated regularly for progression to dementia. Screening instruments (eg. Mini Mental State Examination), neuropsychologic batteries, brief focused cognitive instruments, and structured informant interviews are useful for assessing degree of cognitive impairment.		http://www.aan.com http://www.americangeriatrics.org Neurology 2001;56:1133–1142

DEMENTIA

[a]Triggers that should initiate an assessment for dementia include difficulties in (1) learning and retaining new information, (2) handling complex tasks (eg, balancing a checkbook or cooking a meal), (3) reasoning ability (eg, a new disregard for social norms), (4) spatial ability and orientation (eg, difficulty driving, or getting lost), (5) language (eg, difficulties in word-finding), and (6) behavior (eg, appearing more passive or more irritable than usual).

[b]DSM-IV diagnosis of dementia requires: (1) evidence of decline in functional abilities and (2) evidence of multiple cognitive deficiencies.

[c]See Mini Mental State Examination in Appendix I.

[d]MCI criteria: memory complaint, preferably corroborated by an informant; objective memory impairment; normal general cognitive function; intact activities of daily living; not demented. 6%–25% of MCI patients progress to dementia each year.

Disease Screening	Organization	Date	Population	Recommendations	Comments	Source
DEPRESSION						
Depression	AAFP USPSTF	2003 2002	Children and adolescents	Insufficient evidence to recommend for or against routine screening.	1. Clues to depression include poor school performance, alcohol or drug use, and deteriorating parental or peer relationships. 2. Clues to suicide risk include family dysfunction, physical and sexual abuse, substance abuse, history of recurrent or severe depression, and prior suicide attempt or plans.[a]	
	Bright Futures	2002	Adolescents	Annual screening for behaviors or emotions that might indicate depression or risk of suicide.		
	AAFP USPSTF	2003 2002	Adults	Recommend (but not strongly) screening adults for depression. Screen adults in practices that have systems in place to assure accurate diagnosis, effective treatment, and follow-up.	1. See screening instruments [Geriatric Depression Scale, Beck Depression Inventory (Short Form), PRIME-MD] in Appendix I. 2. Asking 2 simple questions may be as effective as longer instruments (see Appendix I, Screening Tests for Depression). (J Gen Intern Med 1997;12:439) • Over the past 2 weeks, have you felt down, depressed, or hopeless? • Over the past 2 weeks, have you felt little interest or pleasure in doing things? 3. Optimal screening interval is unknown.	http://www.ahrq.gov/clinic/cpgsix.htm

[a]Suicide risk increases as the number of conditions increases. Parents of adolescents at risk for suicide should reduce access to firearms, weapons, or potentially lethal drugs in the home.

Disease Screening	Organization	Date	Population	Recommendations	Comments	Source
Diabetes Mellitus, Gestational (GDM)	ADA	2004	Pregnant women	Risk assess all women. If clinical characteristics consistent with a *high risk* of GDM,[a] do glucose testing at first prenatal visit. If no GDM at initial testing, retest between 24–28 weeks' gestation. *Average-risk women:* test at 24–28 weeks' gestation. *Low-risk women*[b]: no glucose testing.	1. High-quality evidence that asymptomatic screening (vs. testing women with symptoms) for GDM substantially reduces important adverse health outcomes for mothers or their infants is lacking. 2. Fasting plasma glucose >126 mg/dL or a casual plasma glucose > 200 mg/dL meets threshold for diabetes diagnosis, if confirmed on a subsequent day, and precludes the need for glucose challenge. (ADA) 3. Positive 1-hour OGTT: serum glucose > 140 mg/dL after 50 g oral glucose 4. Confirmation test: 3-hour OGTT	Diabetes Care 2004;27(Suppl):S88
	AAFP USPSTF	2003 2003	Pregnant women	Evidence is insufficient to recommend for or against screening.		
	ACOG	2001	Pregnant women	Screen all pregnant women for GDM by patient history, clinical risk factors, and laboratory test.		http://www.acog.org

Disease Screening	Organization	Date	Population	Recommendations	Comments	Source
Diabetes Mellitus, Type 2	ADA	2004	Adults	Consider screening with fasting glucose at 3-year intervals beginning at age 45; consider testing earlier or more frequently in overweight patients if diabetes risk factors present.[c]	1. Cost effectiveness analysis suggests that universal screening is very costly ($360,966 per QALY), in contrast to targeted screening of hypertensives ($34,375 per QALY). (Ann Intern Med 2004;140:689) 2. Impaired fasting glucose: ≥ 110 and < 126 mg/dL. 3. Impaired glucose tolerance: 2 hour PG ≥ 140 and < 200 g/dL. 4. Diabetes defined as fasting glucose ≥ 126 mg/dL on 2 separate occasions, or symptoms of diabetes with random glucose ≥ 200 mg/dL. 5. It has not been demonstrated that beginning diabetes control early as a result of screening provides an incremental benefit compared with initiating treatment after clinical diagnosis. (USPSTF) 6. In hypertensives, there is strong evidence that more aggressive blood pressure control is beneficial when diabetes is present. 7. In hyperlipidemia, NCEP III recommends different treatment thresholds and targets when diabetes is present.	Diabetes Care 2004;27 (Suppl 1):S5
	USPSTF	2003	Adults	Evidence is insufficient to recommend for or against screening asymptomatic adults for type 2 diabetes, impaired glucose tolerance, or impaired fasting glucose.		
	USPSTF	2003	Hypertensive or hyperlipidemic adults	Recommends screening (test and frequency not known).		

[a]High risk is defined as (1) obesity (BMI > 27 kg/m[2]) (see BMI Conversion Table in Appendix IV), (2) strong family history of diabetes, (3) personal history of GDM, or (4) glycosuria.
[b]Low risk for GDM (may *not* need lab screening): < 25 years old; not of Hispanic, African, Native American, South or East Asian, or Pacific Islands ancestry; weight normal before pregnancy; no history of abnormal glucose tolerance; no previous history of poor obstetric outcome; no known diabetes in first-degree relative.
[c]Risk factors (in addition to age ≥45 years) include (1) family history of diabetes in parents or siblings; (2) membership in one of the following ethnic groups: African-American, Hispanic-American, Native American, Asian American, or Pacific Islander; (3) history of impaired fasting glucose, impaired glucose tolerance, gestational diabetes, or mother with infant birthweight > 9 lb; (4) comorbid conditions, including hypertension (> 140/90 mm Hg) or dyslipidemia (HDL < 35 mg/dL or TGs > 250 mg/dL); (5) overweight (BMI ≥ 25 kg/m[2]); (6) polycystic ovary syndrome; and (7) history of vascular disease.

	DOMESTIC VIOLENCE & ABUSE					
Disease Screening	Organization	Date	Population	Recommendations	Comments	Source
Domestic (Intimate Partner) Violence & Abuse	USPSTF	2004	Women Elderly	Insufficient evidence to recommend before or against routine screening	1. Controversy exists regarding the overall benefit of mandatory reporting of domestic violence. (JAMA 1995;273:1781) 2. Barriers to screening include lack of provider education and time. Interventions that incorporated strategies in addition to provider education (eg, providing specific screening questions) were associated with significant increases in identification rates. (Am J Prev Med 2000;19:230) 3. Some states have mandatory reporting of elder abuse and neglect.	Ann Fam Med 2004;2:156
	ACOG	1996	Women	Recommend routine, direct questions about domestic violence[a]		http://www.acog.org

[a]Recommended questions: (1) Within the past year—or since you have been pregnant—have you been hit, slapped, kicked, or otherwise physically hurt by someone?; (2) Are you in a relationship with a person who threatens or physically hurts you?; (3) Has anyone forced you to have sexual activities that made you feel uncomfortable?

FALLS IN THE ELDERLY

Disease Screening	Organization	Date	Population	Recommendations	Comments	Source
Falls in the Elderly	AAOS AGS British Geriatrics Society	2001	All older persons	Ask at least yearly about falls.[a]	1. See also page 70 for fall prevention and Appendix II.	JAGS 2001;49:664–672
	USPSTF	1996	All persons aged ≥ 75 years and those aged 70–74 years with a known risk factor[b]	Counsel about specific measures to prevent falls.		

[a]All who report a single fall should be observed as they stand up from a chair without using their arms, walk several paces, and return (see Appendix II). Those demonstrating no difficulty or unsteadiness need no further assessment. Those who have difficulty or demonstrate unsteadiness, have ≥ 1 fall, or present for medical attention after a fall should have a fall evaluation (see Fall Prevention, page 70).

[b]Risk factors: Intrinsic: lower extremity weakness, poor grip strength, balance disorders, functional and cognitive impairment, visual deficits. Extrinsic: polypharmacy (≥ 4 prescription medications), environment (poor lighting, loose carpets, lack of bathroom safety equipment).

Disease Screening	Organization	Date	Population	Recommendations	Comments	Source
Hearing Impairment	AAP Bright Futures Joint Committee on Infant Hearing[a]	2002 2000 2000	Infants	The hearing of all infants should be screened using objective, physiologic measures to identify those with congenital or neonatal-onset hearing loss.	1. Audiologic evaluations should be in progress before 3 months of age. 2. Infants with confirmed hearing loss should receive intervention before 6 months of age. 3. The efficacy of universal newborn hearing screening to improve long-term language outcomes remains uncertain. (JAMA 2001;286:2000–2010)	Pediatrics 2000;106(4):798–817 http://www.aap.org
	AAFP USPSTF	2003 2001	Normal-risk infants and children	Insufficient evidence to recommend for or against routine screening of neonates. Routine screening beyond age 3 years is not recommended.		http://www.aafp.org/exam.xml http://www.ahrq.gov/clinic/cpgsix.htm
	AAP Bright Futures USPSTF Joint Committee on Infant Hearing[a]	2003 2002 2000 1996	High-risk infants and children[b,c]	Infants should be screened no later than 3 months of age. Screen infants and children < 2 years of age with increased risk. Screen every 6 months until 3 years of age and at appropriate intervals thereafter if there is risk for delayed-onset hearing loss.		Pediatrics 2000;106(4):798–817 http://www.aap.org Pediatrics 2002;111:436–440
	AAP ASHA	2003 1994	High-risk children[c]	Children with frequent recurrent otitis media or middle-ear effusion, or both, should have audiology screening and monitoring of communication-skills development.		http://www.aap.org http://www.asha.org Pediatrics 2003;11:436–440

HEARING IMPAIRMENT

Disease Screening	Organization	Date	Population	Recommendations	Comments	Source
Hearing Impairment (continued)	Bright Futures	2002	Adolescents	Assess annually; screen with objective method at age 12 or more frequently if indicated.		
	AAFP AGS USPSTF CTF	2002 1997 1997 1994	Adults	Question older adults periodically about hearing impairment, counsel about availability of hearing-aid devices, and make referrals for abnormalities when appropriate.	1. Older adults can be screened for hearing loss using simple methods.[d] (JAMA 2003;289:1976–1985)	http://www.aafp.org/exam.xml http://www.ctfphc.org J Am Geriatr Soc 1997;45:344

[a]Joint Committee on Infant Hearing member organizations: American Academy of Audiology; American Academy of Otolaryngology–Head and Neck Surgery; American Academy of Pediatrics; American Speech-Language-Hearing Association; Council on Education of the Deaf; and Directors of Speech and Hearing Programs in State Health and Welfare Agencies.

[b]Increased neonatal risk: family history of hereditary sensorineural hearing loss, intrauterine infection, craniofacial anomalies, birthweight < 1,500 g, hyperbilirubinemia requiring exchange transfusions, ototoxic medications, bacterial meningitis, Apgar scores 0–4 and 0–6, mechanical ventilation lasting > 5 days, and stigmata associated with a syndrome known to include hearing loss.

[c]Increased childhood risk: patient/caregiver concern regarding hearing, speech, language, or developmental delay; bacterial meningitis; head trauma associated with loss of consciousness or skull fracture; stigmata associated with a syndrome known to include hearing loss; ototoxic medications; recurrent or persistent otitis media with effusion; disorders affecting eustachian tube function; neurofibromatosis type 2; and neurodegenerative disorders. Delayed-onset hearing loss: as above for increased childhood risk plus family history of hereditary childhood hearing loss and intrauterine infection.

[d]See also Appendix II: Functional Assessment Screening in the Elderly.

HEPATITIS B VIRUS INFECTION, CHRONIC

Disease Screening	Organization	Date	Population	Recommendations	Comments	Source
Hepatitis B Virus Infection, Chronic	USPSTF CDC	2004 2002	Pregnant women	Screen all women with HBsAg[a] at first prenatal visit. Repeat in third trimester if woman is initially HBsAg negative and engages in high-risk behavior.[b]	1. Screening all pregnant women in the United States each year is estimated to detect 22,000 HBsAg-positive mothers, and treatment of their newborns would prevent chronic HBV infection in 6,000 neonates per year. (Pediatr Infect Dis J 1992;11:866)	MMWR 1991;40(RR-13):1 Int J Gynaecol Obstet 1993;40:172
	USPSTF	2004	General population	Routine screening is not recommended.	1. Most people who become infected as adults recover fully from HBV infection and develop protective immunity. 2. Screening high-risk persons[b] would still miss 30%–40% of cases.	

[a]Immunoassays for HBsAg have sensitivity and specificity > 98%. (MMWR 1993;42:707)
[b]High risk includes injection drug users, sexual contact with HBV-infected persons or with persons at high risk for HBV infection, multiple sexual partners, and male homosexual activity.

HEPATITIS C VIRUS INFECTION, CHRONIC

Disease Screening	Organization	Date	Population	Recommendations	Comments	Source
Hepatitis C Virus Infection, Chronic	USPSTF	2004	General population	Do not perform routine screening for HCV infection in adults who are not at increased risk.[a]	1. 15%–25% of persons with acute hepatitis C resolve their infection; of the remaining, 10%–20% develop cirrhosis within 20–30 years after infection, and 1%–5% develop hepatocellular carcinoma. 2. Abstinence from alcohol is imperative in patients with chronic hepatitis C.	
	USPSTF	2004	Persons at increased risk[a]	Insufficient evidence to recommend for or against routine screening.	3. Although antiviral therapy can improve intermediate outcomes, such as viremia, there is limited evidence that such treatment improves long-term outcomes. 4. Potential harms of screening include unnecessary biopsies and labeling, as well as adverse effects of antiviral therapy.	MWMR 2003;52(RR-1) Pediatrics 1998;101(3):481
	CDC AAP	2003 1998	Persons at increased risk[a]	Perform routine counseling, testing, and appropriate follow-up.[b] See algorithm on page 43.		

[a] Increased risk includes injection drug use, receipt of clotting factor concentrates before 1987, chronic hemodialysis, persistently abnormal alanine aminotransferase levels, receipt of blood from a donor who later tested positive for HCV, receipt of blood transfusion or blood components before July 1992, receipt of organ transplant before July 1992, health care workers after needle sticks or mucosal exposures to HCV-positive blood, and children born to HCV-positive women.
[b] 3 types of tests are available for laboratory diagnosis of HCV infection: (1) detection of antibody to HCV antigens, and (2) detection and quantification of HCV nucleic acid. See algorithm on page 43.

HCV INFECTION TESTING ALGORITHM FOR ASYMPTOMATIC PERSONS

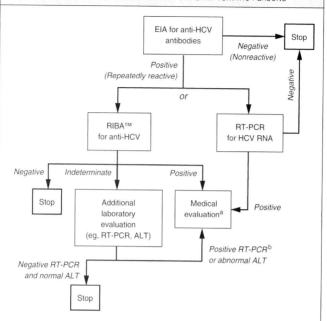

ALT = alanine aminotransferase; anti-HCV = antibody to HCV; EIA = enzyme immunoassay; RIBA™ = recombinant immunoblot assay; RT-PCR = reverse transcriptase polymerase chain reaction

[a]For possible anti-inflammatory and antiviral treatments.

[b]Treatment with combination peg-interferon alfa-2b plus ribavirin leads to sustained virologic response in about 50% of patients with detectable HCV RNA **and** elevated ALT. (Lancet 2001;358:958) Some liver disease specialists recommend liver biopsy and appropriate treatment in all patients with detectable HCV RNA, regardless of ALT levels. (Hepatology 2001;33:196)

Source: Adapted from MMWR 1998;47(RR-19):1.

HUMAN IMMUNODEFICIENCY VIRUS					
Disease Screening	**Organization**	**Date**	**Population**	**Recommendations**	**Comments**	**Source**

Disease Screening	Organization	Date	Population	Recommendations	Comments	Source
Human Immunodeficiency Virus	AAFP	2003	Infants born to high-risk mothers[a]	Recommends (not strongly) screening.	1. Protect client confidentiality and be voluntary with informed consent. Provide patients with option for anonymous testing, written materials about HIV testing. 2. HIV prevention counseling focuses on client's own risk.	http://www.aafp.org/exam.xml
	AAFP	2003	People at increased risk[a]	Strongly recommends screening.	3. Initial screening test: EIA is considered reactive only when a positive result is confirmed in a second test of the original sample. Seroconversion is 95% within 6 months of infection. Specificity is > 99.5%.	http://www.aafp.org/exam.xml
	CDC	2001	People at increased risk[a]	Routine and targeted counseling, testing, and referral (CTR) for HIV disease should be based on type of clinical setting, HIV prevalence in setting, and behavioral and clinical risk of individual clients in the setting.	4. False-positives with EIA: nonspecific reactions in persons with immunologic disturbances (eg, systemic lupus erythematosus or rheumatoid arthritis), multiple transfusions, recent influenza, or rabies vaccination. 5. Confirmatory testing is necessary using Western blot or indirect immunofluorescence assay. 6. Home tests available.[b]	MMWR 2001;50(RR-19):1

HUMAN IMMUNODEFICIENCY VIRUS					
Disease Screening	Organization	Date	Population	Recommendations	Comments	Source
Human Immunodeficiency Virus (continued)	AAFP CDC ACOG	2001 2001 2000	Pregnant women	Universal testing with patient notification of all pregnant women (ie, testing is routinely performed unless patient actively refuses). Consent to testing should be in writing. Retest high-risk women at 36 weeks' gestation.	1. Pretest counseling modified to alleviate this burdensome barrier to testing as recommended by the Institute of Medicine Report. 2. HIV testing as a routine part of antenatal care increased screening rates from 75% to 88%. (Obstet Gynecol 2001;98:1104) 3. Rapid HIV antibody testing during labor identified 34 positive women among 4,849 women with no prior HIV testing documented (prevalence, 7 in 1,000). 84% of women consented to testing. Sensitivity was 100%, specificity was 99.9%, PPV was 90%. (JAMA 2004;292:219)	MMWR 2001;50(RR-19);59 Pediatrics 1995;95:303 NEJM 1994;331:1173 http://www.aafp.org/exam.xml

HUMAN IMMUNODEFICIENCY VIRUS

[a]High risk: seeking treatment for STDs; male homosexual sex after 1975; past or current exchange of sex for money or drugs; sex partners of people who are HIV-infected, bisexual, or injection drug users; or history of blood transfusion between 1978 and 1985.

[b]The FDA has approved 2 HIV home testing kits and warns about use of HIV home testing kits that have not been FDA approved. Consumers can obtain information about HIV home testing kits by calling the HIV/AIDS Program of the FDA in the Office of Special Health Issues at 301-827-4460. Health care provider follow-up is recommended for positive home HIV test results. [Oncology 1999;13(1):81]

EIA = enzyme immunoassay

HYPERTENSION, CHILDREN & ADOLESCENTS					
Disease Screening	Organization	Date	Population	Recommendations	Comments	Source
Hypertension, Children & Adolescents	USPSTF	2003	Aged < 21 years	Insufficient evidence to recommend for or against routine screening	1. Hypertension: BP > 95th percentile 3 different times within 1 month, adjusted for height. (J Pediatr 1993;123:871) (see Appendix III) 2. Major reason to screen children is early identification of conditions associated with hypertension (eg, coarctation of aorta, renal artery stenosis, renal parenchymal disease). 3. Treatment of primary (essential) hypertension in older children and adolescents is of unproved benefit; the majority respond to weight loss and exercise.[a] (Am J Cardiol 1983;52:763, Pediatrics 1978;61:245)	Pediatrics 1987;79:1 Pediatrics 1996;98:649
	NHLBI	1996	Aged 3–20 years	Annual screening		
	Bright Futures	1994	Aged 3–21 years	Annual screening at ages 3–6, 8, and 10–21 years		
	GAPS	1994	Aged 11–18 years	Annual screening		

Disease Screening	Organization	Date	Population	Recommendations	Comments	Source
Hypertension, Adults	British Hypertension Society	2004	Aged 18–80 years	Screen at least every 5 years If SBP > 130 or DBP > 85, then annually		BMJ 2004;328:634–640
	JNC VII (NHLBI)	2003	Aged > 18 years	Normal: recheck in 2 years (see Comments) Prehypertension: recheck in 1 year Stage 1 hypertension: confirm within 2 months Stage 2 hypertension: evaluate or refer to source of care within 1 month (evaluate and treat immediately if BP > 180/110)	1. Prehypertension: SBP 120–139 or DBP 80–89 2. Stage 1 hypertension: SBP 140–159 or DBP 90–99 3. Stage 2 hypertension: SBP ≥ 160 or DBP ≥ 100 (based on average of ≥ 2 measurements on ≥ 2 separate office visits) 4. Finger monitors are not accurate. [Fam Med 1996;61(50):53] 5. Perform physical exam and routine labs.[b] 6. Pursue secondary causes of hypertension.[c] 7. Treatment goals are for BP < 140/90, unless diabetes or renal disease present (< 130/80). See JNC VII Management Algorithm, page 117. 8. Ambulatory BP monitoring is a better (and independent) predictor of cardiovascular outcomes compared with office visit monitoring.	JAMA 2003;289:2560 Hypertension 2003;42:1206–1252
	USPSTF	2003	Aged ≥ 18 years	Strongly recommends screening		Hypertension 2000;35:844 NEJM 2003;348:2407–2415
	AAFP	2002	Aged > 21 years	Strongly recommends periodic screening If SBP < 140/85 mm Hg, then every 2 years If DBP 85–89 mm Hg, then annually		http://www.aafp.org/exam.xml

HYPERTENSION, ADULTS

[a]The NHLBI recommends pharmacologic treatment of severe hypertension in addition to nonpharmacologic treatment (< 1% of hypertensive children are classified as severe). (Arch Dis Child 1967;42:34)

[b]Physical exam should include: measurements of height, weight, and waist circumference; funduscopic exam (retinopathy); carotid auscultation (bruit); jugular venous pulsation; thyroid gland (enlargement); cardiac auscultation (left ventricular heave, S_3 or S_4 murmurs, clicks); chest auscultation (rales, evidence of chronic obstructive pulmonary disease); abdominal exam (bruits, masses, pulsations); exam of lower extremities (diminished arterial pulsations, bruits, edema); and neurologic exam (focal findings). Routine labs include urinalysis, complete blood count, electrolytes (potassium, calcium), creatinine, glucose, fasting lipids, and 12-lead electrocardiogram.

[c]Pursue secondary causes of hypertension when evaluation is suggestive (clues in parentheses) of: (1) pheochromocytoma (labile or paroxysmal hypertension accompanied by sweats, headaches, and palpitations), (2) renovascular disease (abdominal bruits), (3) autosomal dominant polycystic kidney disease (abdominal or flank masses), (4) Cushing's syndrome (truncal obesity with purple striae), (5) primary hyperaldosteronism (hypokalemia), (6) hyperparathyroidism (hypercalcemia), (7) renal parenchymal disease (elevated serum creatinine, abnormal urinalysis), (8) poor response to drug therapy, (9) well-controlled hypertension with an abrupt increase in blood pressure, (10) SBP > 180 or DBP > 110 mm Hg, or (11) sudden onset of hypertension.

LEAD POISONING

Disease Screening	Organization	Date	Population	Recommendations	Comments	Source
Lead Poisoning	ACPM	2001	Infants and children	Selective screening at 12 months for infants and children at high risk[a]	1. Risk assessment should be performed during prenatal visits and continuing until 6 years of age. 2. CDC personal risk questionnaire: (1) Does your child live in or regularly visit a house (or other facility, eg, daycare) that was built before 1950? (2) Does your child live in or regularly visit a house built before 1978 with recent or ongoing renovations or remodeling (within the last 6 months)? (3) Does your child have a sibling or playmate who has or did have lead poisoning?	Am J Prev Med 2001;20:78
	CDC AAP	2000 1998	Infants and children	Selective screening with blood lead level at 9–12 months, and again at 24 months when levels peak, of infants and children at high risk[a] Evaluation of blood lead level[b]		Pediatrics 1998;101:1072 http://www.cdc.gov/ mmwr/pdf/rr/rr4914.pdf
	AAFP USPSTF	2001 1996	Infants at age 12 months	Selective screening with blood lead level for those infants at high risk[a]		http://www.aafp.org/ exam.xml

[a]Criteria for being at high risk include: receipt of Medicaid or WIC; living in a community with ≥ 12% prevalence of elevated blood lead levels (BLLs) at ≥ 10 μg/mL; living in a community with ≥ 27% of homes built before 1950; or meeting 1 or more high risk criteria from a lead-screening questionnaire (see CDC comments in table). Prevalence levels supported by recent cost-effectiveness studies. (Arch Pediatr Adolesc Med 1998;152:1202) Additional criteria: living near lead industry or heavy traffic or living with someone whose job or hobby involves lead exposure or who uses lead-based pottery or takes traditional remedies that contain lead.
[b]Confirm elevated lead levels with venous sample after screening sample from fingerstick: immediately if > 70 μg/mL, within 48 hours if 45–69 μg/mL, within 1 week if 20–44 μg/mL, and within 1 month if 10–19 μg/mL. See AAP guidelines for further treatment recommendations.

Disease Screening	Organization	Date	Population	Recommendations	Comments	Source
OBESITY						
Obesity	AAP	2003	Children and adolescents	Calculate and plot BMI annually.	1. Overweight is defined as BMI 25–29.9 kg/m^2 and obesity as BMI > 30 kg/m^2.	Pediatrics 2003;112:424–430
	NHLBI	2000	Age > 18 years	Calculate BMI and measure waist circumference for all patients.[a]	2. The NHLBI makes a strong case for promoting weight loss in overweight individuals, particularly those with hypertension, diabetes, cardiovascular disease, and hyperlipidemia. 3. Waist–hip ratio may also provide additional prognostic information beyond BMI and waist circumference. Among women 50–69 years of age free of cancer, heart disease, and diabetes, waist–hip ratio is the best anthropometric predictor of total mortality. (Arch Intern Med 2000;160:2117)	NHLBI Obesity Guidelines in Adults, 1998 NHLBI. The Practical Guide: Identification, Evaluation, and Treatment of Overweight and Obesity in Adults, 2000
	AAFP USPSTF Maternal and Child Health Bureau	2003 2003 1998	All age groups	Periodic height and weight measurements.	4. In July 2004, Centers for Medicare and Medicaid Services dropped language that had resulted in routine denial of coverage for weight-loss therapies. Agency will review scientific evidence for therapies to determine coverage. (http://www.washingtonpost.com, accessed July 23, 2004)	http://www.aafp.org/exam.xml

[a]BMI is calculated as: weight (kg)/height (m) squared. See Appendix IV for BMI Conversion Table. Studies do not support a BMI range of 25–27 as a risk factor for all-cause and cardiovascular mortality among elderly (age ≥ 65 years) persons. (Arch Intern Med 2001;161:1194) BMI cut-offs may also need to be modified for some Asian populations. (http://www.idi.org.au; Am J Clin Nutr 2001;73:123)

OSTEOPOROSIS

Disease Screening	Organization	Date	Population	Recommendations	Comments	Source
Osteoporosis	ACOG AACE AAFP NOF USPSTF	2004 2003 2003 2002 2002	Women aged ≥ 65 years	Routine[a] screening of bone mineral density (BMD)	1. The benefits of screening and treatment are of at least moderate magnitude for women at ↑ risk by virtue of age or presence of other risk factors.[a] 2. Dual energy x-ray absorptiometry is the most accurate clinical method for identifying those with low BMD.	http://www.acog.org http://www.nof.org Ann Intern Med 2002;137:526 http://www.aace.com/clin/guidelines
	ACOG AACE AAFP NOF USPSTF	2004 2003 2003 2002 2002	Women at increased risk for osteoporotic fractures[a,b,c]	Routine[a] screening beginning at age 60.	3. The Simple Calculated Osteoporosis Risk Estimation (SCORE) and Osteoporosis Risk Assessment Instrument (ORAI) decision rules are better than NOF guidelines at targeting BMD testing in high-risk patients. (JAMA 2001;286:57–63) 4. Refer to osteoporosis screening algorithm on page 53.	http://www.acog.org http://www.nof.org Ann Intern Med 2002;137:526 http://www.aace.com/clin/guidelines

[a]AACE recommends follow-up BMD measure in 3–5 years for women with "normal" baseline score, and if high risk, in 1–2 years.

[b]Exact risk factors that should trigger screening in this age group are difficult to specify based on evidence. Well-accepted high-risk factors include chronic steroid use (≥ 2 months), repeated fractures or fractures not caused by trauma, early menopause, low body weight (< 127 lb), cigarette use.

[c]See table of risk factors on page 54.

OSTEOPOROSIS: SCREENING

SELECTIVE SCREENING FOR OSTEOPOROSIS IN PERSONS NOT
CURRENTLY TAKING ANTI-OSTEOPOROSIS
MEDICATIONS OR HAVING A HISTORY OF HIP FRACTURE
(Modified from the National Osteoporosis Foundation:
Physician's guide to prevention & treatment of osteoporosis;
Up To Date Screening for Osteoporosis by H.N. Rosen).

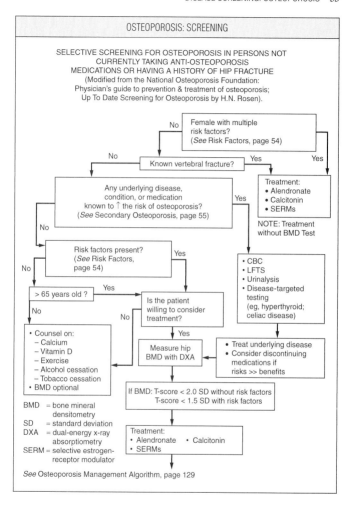

BMD = bone mineral densitometry
SD = standard deviation
DXA = dual-energy x-ray absorptiometry
SERM = selective estrogen-receptor modulator

See Osteoporosis Management Algorithm, page 129

RISK FACTORS FOR OSTEOPOROTIC FRACTURE	
Potentially Modifiable	**Nonmodifiable**
Current cigarette smoker	*Personal history of fracture as an adult*
Low body weight (< 127 lb)	*History of fracture in first-degree relative*
Estrogen deficiency: -early menopause (age < 45 years) or bilateral ovariectomy -prolonged premenopausal amenorrhea (> 1 year)	Caucasian race
Low calcium intake (lifelong)	Advanced age
Alcohol (> 2 drinks/day)	Female sex
Impaired eyesight despite adequate correction	Dementia
Recurrent falls	
Inadequate physical activity	
Poor health/frailty	

Italicized items—personal or family history of fracture, smoking, and low body weight—were demonstrated in a large, ongoing, prospective U.S. study to be key factors in determining the risk of hip fracture (independent of bone density).
Source: National Osteoporosis Foundation.
Physician's guide to prevention and treatment of osteoporosis. Available at: http://www.nof.org/physguide, accessed December 12, 2003.

Drugs	Endocrine Diseases or Metabolic Causes	Collagen Vascular Diseases	Nutritional Conditions	Other Causes
	CAUSES OF GENERALIZED SECONDARY OSTEOPOROSIS IN ADULTS			
Aluminum	Acromegaly	Epidermolysis bullosa	Gastrectomy	Amyloidosis
Anticonvulsants	Adrenal atrophy and	Osteogenesis	Eating	Ankylosing
Cigarette smoking	Addison's disease	imperfecia	disorders	spondylitis
Cytotoxic drugs	Congenital porphyria		Malabsorption	AIDS/HIV
Excessive alcohol	Cushing's syndrome		syndromes	Chronic
Excessive thyroxine	Endometriosis		Nutritional	obstructive
Glucocorticosteroids &	Female athlete triad		disorders	pulmonary
adrenocorticotropin	Gaucher's disease		Parenteral	disease
(oral or inhaled)	Gonadal		nutrition	Hemophilia
Gonadotropin-	insufficiency		Pernicious	Idiopathic
releasing hormone	(primary &		anemia	scoliosis
agonists	secondary)		Severe liver	Inflammatory
Heparin	Hemochromatosis		disease	bowel
Immune suppressants	Hyperparathyroidism		(especially	disease
Lithium	Hypophosphatemia		primary	Lymphoma &
Tamoxifen	Diabetes mellitus,		biliary	leukemia
(premenopausal use)	type 1		cirrhosis)	Mastocytosis
	Thyrotoxicosis		Sprue	Multiple
	Tumor secretion of			myeloma
	parathyroid			Multiple
	hormone–related			sclerosis
	peptide			Rheumatoid
				arthritis
				Sarcoidosis
				Spinal cord
				transection
				Stroke
				Thalassemia

Source: National Osteoporosis Foundation.
Physician's guide to prevention and treatment of osteoporosis. Available at:
http://www.nof.org/physguide, accessed December 12, 2003.

SCOLIOSIS					
Disease Screening	Organization	Date	Population	Recommendations	Comments	Source
Scoliosis	USPSTF	2004	Adolescents	Recommends against routine screening.	1. Positive predictive value of bending test is 42.8% for scoliosis of > 5 degrees and 6.4% for > 15 degrees; sensitivity 74%, specificity 78%. (Am J Public Health 1985;75:1377)	
	Bright Futures	2002	Adolescents	Screen during physical exam annually in adolescents and children > 8 years of age.		
	AAOS	1992	Adolescents	Screen girls twice (ages 10 and 12 years) and boys once (age 13 or 14 years).		http://www.aaos.org
	Scoliosis Research Society	1986	Adolescents	Perform annual screening of all children aged 10–14 years.		Scoliosis Research Society: Scoliosis: A Handbook for Patients. Scoliosis Research Society, 1986

SYPHILIS

Disease Screening	Organization	Date	Population	Recommendations	Comments	Source
Syphilis	AAFP AAP ACOG USPSTF	2003 1997 1997 1996	Pregnant women	Screen all pregnant women with nontreponemal test (eg, RPR or VDRL) at first prenatal visit; repeat in third trimester and at delivery for women at high risk of acquiring infection during pregnancy.	1. All reactive nontreponemal tests should be confirmed with a more specific treponemal test (eg, FTA-ABS). 2. Perform follow-up serologic tests after treatment to document decline in titers (using the same test used initially). 3. Sensitivity of nontreponemal tests varies with levels of antibodies: 62%–76% in early primary syphilis, 100% during secondary syphilis, and 70% in untreated late syphilis. In late syphilis, previously reactive results revert to nonreactive in 25% of patients. 4. Specificity of nontreponemal tests is 75%–85% in persons with preexisting diseases or conditions (eg, collagen vascular diseases, injection drug use, advanced malignancy, pregnancy, malaria, tuberculosis, viral and rickettsial diseases) and 100% in persons without preexisting diseases or conditions. 5. Syphilis outbreaks have been recently reported among California gay men and Alabama prisoners. (Am J Public Health 2001;91:1220, JAMA 2001;285:1285)	Ann Intern Med 1986;104:368 Pediatrics 1994;94:568 MMWR 1993;42 (RR-14):1 http://www.aafp.org/exam.xml
	AAFP AAP ACOG USPSTF	2003 1997 1997 1996	High-risk persons[a]	Screen high-risk persons with routine serologic test (eg, RPR or VDRL).		
	AAN	2001	Patients with dementia	Do not screen unless clinical suspicion of neurosyphilis is present.		Neurology 2001;56:1143

[a]High risk includes commercial sex workers, persons who exchange sex for money or drugs, persons with other STDs (including HIV), and sexual contacts of persons with active syphilis.

Disease Screening	Organization	Date	Population	Recommendations	Comments	Source
Thyroid Disease	USPSTF AAFP	2004 2003	Children and adults	Routine screening is not recommended.	1. Increased risk of hypothyroidism among patients with autoimmune diseases, unexplained depression, cognitive dysfunction, or hypercholesterolemia.	Ann Intern Med 2004;140:125–127 http://www.aafp.org/exam.xml
	ATA	2000	Women aged ≥ 35 years	Screen with serum TSH at age 35 years, and every 5 years thereafter.	2. Individuals with symptoms and signs potentially attributable to thyroid dysfunction[a] and those with risk factors for its development[b] may require more frequent TSH testing.	Arch Intern Med 2000;160:1573
	ACP	1998	Women aged > 50 years	Perform selective screening for women with 1 or more general symptoms such as fatigue, weight gain, or depression.	3. When there is suspicion of pituitary or hypothalamic disease, the serum FT4 concentration should be measured in addition to the serum TSH. 4. Clinicians should remain alert for subtle or nonspecific symptoms of hypothyroidism and maintain a low threshold for diagnostic evaluation using serum TSH.	Ann Intern Med 1998;129:141–143
	AACE	2002	Elderly	Periodic screening with sensitive TSH.	5. Controversy exists regarding Rx benefit for patients with subclinical hypothyroidism (elevated TSH; normal free thyroxine).	http://www.aace.com/clin/guidelines Endocrine Practice 2002;8:457–469

[a]Signs, symptoms, and comorbidities suggestive of hypothyroidism include previous thyroid dysfunction, goiter, surgery or radiotherapy affecting the thyroid, diabetes mellitus, vitiligo, pernicious anemia, leukotrichia (prematurely gray hair), and medications (such as lithium carbonate and iodine-containing compounds, eg, amiodarone, radiocontrast agents, expectorants containing potassium iodide, and kelp).

[b]Risk factors include family history of thyroid disease, or personal history of pernicious anemia, diabetes mellitus, and primary adrenal insufficiency. Laboratory test results suggestive of thyroid disease include hypercholesterolemia, hyponatremia, anemia, CPK and LDH elevations, hyperprolactinemia, hypercalcemia, alkaline phosphatase elevation, and hepatocellular enzyme elevation.

THYROID DISEASE

Disease Screening	Organization	Date	Population	Recommendation	Comments	Source
TOBACCO USE						
Tobacco Use	USPSTF	2003	Children and adolescents	Evidence is insufficient to recommend for or against routine screening.		
	USPSTF	2003	Adults	Screen for tobacco use. See treatment algorithm on page 146.	1. Smoking cessation lowers the risk of heart disease, stroke, and lung disease.	
	USPSTF	2003	Pregnant women	Screen for tobacco use.	1. Extended or augmented counseling (5–15 minutes) that is tailored for pregnant smokers is more effective (17% abstinence) than generic counseling (7% abstinence). 2. Cessation leads to increased birth weights.	

						TUBERCULOSIS
Disease Screening	Organization	Date	Population	Recommendations	Comments	Source
Tuberculosis	ATS CDC AAFP Bright Futures USPSTF	2003 2003 2002 2002 1996	Persons at increased risk of developing TB[a]	Screening by tuberculin skin test is recommended.[b] Frequency of testing should be based on likelihood of further exposure to TB and level of confidence in the accuracy of the results.[c]	1. Persons with positive PPD test should receive chest x-ray and clinical evaluation for TB. If no evidence of active infection, provide INH prophylaxis if appropriate. 2. The purpose of targeted testing is to find and treat persons who have both latent TB infection *and high risk for reactivation of TB*. Persons with ≥ 10 mm induration on PPD test and who have either HIV infection or evidence of old, healed TB have the highest lifetime risk of reactivation (≥ 20%). Also at high risk (10%–20%) are those with 1) recent PPD conversion, 2) age > 35 years and immunosuppressive therapy, and 3) induration > 15 mm and age < 35 years. (NEJM 2004;350:2060) Thus, consider retesting persons with history of positive PPD of unknown induration. 3. Treatment (INH for 9 months) is recommended for foreign-born persons from countries with a high prevalence of TB who have latent TB infection and who have been in the United States < 5 years. 4. Prior BCG vaccination is not considered a valid basis for dismissing positive results. 5. Because sporadic INH-associated liver injury still occurs, patients taking INH should be monitored as indicated (history of liver disorder, HIV infection, pregnant and immediate post-partum women, regular alcohol user). [MMWR 2001;50(34)]	http://www.aafp.org/exam.xml MMWR 2003;52(RR-02);15–18 MMWR 2000;49(RR-06);1–54

TUBERCULOSIS

[a]Increased risk: persons infected with HIV, close contacts of persons with known or suspected TB (including health care workers), persons with medical risk factors associated with reactivation of TB (eg, silicosis, diabetes mellitus, prolonged corticosteroid therapy, end-stage renal disease, immunosuppressive therapy), immigrants from countries with high TB prevalence (eg, most countries in Africa, Asia, and Latin America), medically underserved and low-income populations, alcoholics, injection drug users, persons with abnormal CXRs compatible with past TB, and residents of long-term care facilities (eg, correctional institutions, mental institutions, nursing homes).

[b]Test: Give intradermal injection of 5 U of tuberculin PPD and examine 48–72 hours later. Criteria for positive skin test (diameter of induration): > 15 mm for low risk, > 10 mm for high risk (including children < 4 years of age), > 5 mm for very high risk (HIV, abnormal CXR, recent contact with infected persons). If negative, consider 2-step testing to differentiate between booster effect and new conversion. Perform second test within 13 weeks. False-negative results occur in 5%–10%, especially early in infection, with anergy, with concurrent severe illness, in newborns and infants < 3 months old, and with improper technique.

[c]Periodic (eg, at ages 1, 4–6, and 6–11 years) tuberculin skin testing is recommended for children who live in high-prevalence regions or whose history for risk factors is incomplete or unreliable.

VISUAL IMPAIRMENT, GLAUCOMA, & CATARACT

Disease Screening	Organization	Date	Population	Recommendations	Comments	Source
Visual Impairment, Glaucoma, & Cataract	AAP	2003	Infants and children[a]	Assess for eye problems in the newborn period and then at all subsequent routine health supervision visits. Visual acuity testing beginning at age 3 years.		Opthalmology 2003;110:860–865 Pediatrics 2003;111:902–907
	AOA	2002	Infants and children	Initial eye and vision screening at birth, then at age 6 months, age 3 years, and every 2 years thereafter.		http://www.aoanet.org
	USPSTF	2004	Children	Recommends screening to detect amblyopia, strabismus, and defects in visual acuity before age 5 years.		
	AAFP	2003	Children	Vision screening for amblyopia and strabismus between ages 3 and 4 years.		http://www.aafp.org/exam.xml
	AAO	2000	Adults	Comprehensive eye and vision exam every 3–5 years in blacks aged 20–39 years, and, regardless of race, every 2–4 years aged 40–64 years and every 1–2 years beginning age 65 years.		http://www.aao.org
	AOA	1997	Adults	Comprehensive eye and vision exam every 2–3 years aged 18–40 years, every 2 years aged 41–60 years, and every 1 year aged ≥ 61 years.		http://www.aoanet.org

VISUAL IMPAIRMENT, GLAUCOMA, & CATARACT					
Disease Screening	Organization	Date	Population	Recommendations	Comments	Source
Visual Impairment, Glaucoma, & Cataract (continued)	USPSTF	1996	Adults	Insufficient evidence to recommend routine eye and vision screening or screening for elevated intraocular pressure or glaucoma by primary care physicians among asymptomatic nonelderly adults.		
	AAFP AGS USPSTF CTF	2003 1997 1996 1995	Elderly	Perform routine eye and Snellen visual acuity screening. Optimal frequency is not known.		J Am Geriatr Soc 1997;45:344 http://www.aafp.org/exam.xml CMAJ 1995;152:1211–1222

[a]Refer to ophthalmologist if high risk (very premature; family congenital cataracts, retinoblastoma, or metabolic or genetic diseases; significant developmental delay or neurologic difficulties; systemic disease associated with eye abnormalities).

2
Disease Prevention

Disease Prevention	Organization	Date	Population	Recommendations	Comments	Source
Breast Cancer	NCI	2004	Women	Avoid unnecessary breast irradiation. *Genetic screening:* Little evidence to support or quantify potential beneficial effect of genetic screening (*BRCA1/BRCA2*). *SERMs:* Based on good evidence, tamoxifen reduces the incidence of breast cancer in postmenopausal women. Risks and benefits have to be weighed.[a] *Mastectomy:* Because of the physical and psychological effects and the irreversibility of the procedure, decisions regarding this option must be considered on an individual basis.	1. Low-fat diet and exercise may decrease risk. Alcohol and obesity may increase risk. 2. Known genetic syndromes contribute to ~5% of breast cancers. 3. An RCT has shown that tamoxifen reduces the risk of developing breast cancer in women at increased risk. Tamoxifen increases the risk of endometrial cancer and of thrombotic vascular events. (J Natl Cancer Inst 1998;90:1371) 4. Women being considered for tamoxifen therapy should be evaluated by health care providers familiar with evaluation of individual breast cancer risk and the risks and benefits of tamoxifen use. 5. The WHI found that combined estrogen and progestin HRT leads to an increased risk of breast cancer. (JAMA 2003;289) The use of HRT after diagnosis of breast cancer significantly increased the risk for recurrence. (Lancet 2004;363) 6. In retrospective studies, progestin-only contraception was not associated with increased risk of breast cancer. (Contraception 2004;69)	http://www.cancer.gov J Natl Cancer Inst 2001;93(21):1633–1637 NEJM 1999;340(2):77–84
	CTF	2000	Low-/normal-risk women (< 1.66% on Gail index)[b]	Recommend against use of tamoxifen to reduce the risk of breast cancer.		

	BREAST CANCER					

Disease Prevention	Organization	Date	Population	Recommendations	Comments	Source
Breast Cancer (continued)	ASCO CTF	2002 2001	Women at high risk[b]	For women with a 5-year projected risk of breast cancer of ≥ 1.66%, tamoxifen (at 20 mg/day for up to 5 years) may be offered to reduce their risk. Tamoxifen use should be discussed as part of an informed decision-making process, with careful consideration of risks and benefits.[a]	7. Premature to recommend raloxifene, tamoxifen combined with hormone replacement therapy, aromatase inhibitors or inactivators, or femretinide use to lower the risk of developing breast cancer outside of a clinical trial setting.[c] 8. Bilateral prophylactic mastectomy is associated with a reduction in risk of breast cancer by as much as 90% among women with an increased risk of breast cancer due to a strong family history or with BRCA1 or BRCA2 alterations.	http://www.asco.org J Clin Oncol 1999;17(6);1939 CMAJ 2001;164(12);1681–1690

[a]Tamoxifen treatment increases the risk of endometrial cancer, thrombotic vascular events, and cataracts.

[b]Predicted risk of breast cancer calculated by using the Gail model, which considers age, number of first-degree relatives with breast cancer, number of previous breast biopsies, age at first live birth, and age at menarche. (J Natl Cancer Inst 1999;91:1829) The Breast Cancer Risk Assessment Tool allows health professionals to project a woman's individualized estimate of risk for invasive breast cancer over a 5-year period and lifetime. (http://bcra.nci.nih.gov/brc)

[c]Among postmenopausal women with osteoporosis, the risk of invasive breast cancer was decreased by 75% during 3 years of treatment with raloxifene. [JAMA 1999;281(23);2189] The MORE trial found that measurement of estradiol level by sensitive assay in postmenopausal women identifies those at high risk of breast cancer. These women benefited most from reduction in risk of breast cancer with raloxifene treatment. (JAMA 2002;287:216–220) The Study of Tamoxifen and Raloxifene (STAR) began recruiting volunteers in May 1999. This study will compare tamoxifen and raloxifene for their effects on reduction of breast cancer development in postmenopausal women. Information about this and other breast cancer prevention trials is available from http://cancer.gov/star or from the National Cancer Institute's Cancer Information Service (1-800-422-6237). The NCI is conducting the Capital Area SERM study to evaluate the safety of raloxifene in premenopausal women who are at increased risk for breast cancer (1-888-624-1937).

					DIABETES, TYPE 2	
Disease Prevention	Organization	Date	Population	Recommendations	Comments	Source
Diabetes, Type 2	ADA	2003	Patients with impaired fasting glucose or glucose tolerance (see page 36)	Counsel on increasing physical activity and weight loss. Follow-up counseling important for success. Monitor for diabetes every 1–2 years.	1. Drug therapy should not be routinely used to prevent diabetes until more information is known about cost-effectiveness. 2. RCTs have proven the efficacy of increased physical activity and weight loss for preventing type 2 diabetes. (NEJM 2002;346:393) In overweight patients (mean BMI, 34 kg/m^2), nutrition/exercise intervention group had 4.8% incidence of progression to diabetes compared with control group (11.0% incidence).	Diabetes Care 2003;26(Suppl 1):S62

ENDOCARDITIS

Disease Prevention	Organization	Date	Population	Recommendations	Comments	Source
Endocarditis	ASCRS AHA	2000 1997	High-risk persons[a] Moderate-risk persons[b]	Give antibiotic prophylaxis[c] before bacteremia-producing procedures.[d,e]		JAMA 1997;277:1794

[a]Patients at high risk for endocarditis include those with prosthetic heart valves (including bioprosthetic and homograft valves), previous bacterial endocarditis, complex cyanotic congenital heart disease (including single ventricle states, transposition of the great arteries, tetralogy of Fallot), and surgically constructed systemic pulmonary shunts or conduits.

[b]Patients at moderate risk for endocarditis include those with most other congenital heart diseases (excluding isolated secundum atrial septal defect and surgically repaired atrial septal defect, ventricular septal defect, or patent ductus arteriosus without residua beyond 6 months), acquired valvular dysfunction (eg, rheumatic heart disease), hypertrophic cardiomyopathy, and mitral valve prolapse with valvular regurgitation or thickened leaflets.

[c]Standard prophylaxis regimen for dental, oral, respiratory tract, or esophageal procedures: amoxicillin (adults 2.0 g; children 50 mg/kg orally 1 hour before procedure). If unable to take oral medications, give ampicillin (adults 2.0 g IM or IV; children 50 mg/kg IM or IV within 30 minutes of procedure). If penicillin-allergic, give clindamycin (adults 600 mg; children 20 mg/kg orally 1 hour before procedure) or cephalexin or cefadroxil (adults 2.0 g; children 50 mg/kg orally 1 hour before procedure), or azithromycin or clarithromycin (adults 500 mg; children 15 mg/kg orally 1 hour before procedure). If penicillin-allergic and unable to take oral medications, give clindamycin (adults 600 mg; children 20 mg/kg IV within 30 minutes before procedure) or cefazolin (adults 1 g; children 25 mg/kg IM or IV within 30 minutes of procedure). See reference for recommended antibiotic regimens for other procedures. (JAMA 1997;277:1794)

[d]Bacteremia-producing procedures include: (1) dental and oral procedures including dental extractions, periodontal procedures, dental implant placement and reimplantation of avulsed teeth, endodontic (root canal) instrumentation, subgingival placement of antibiotic fibers or strips, initial placement of orthodontic bands but not brackets, intraligamentary local anesthetic injections, and prophylactic cleaning of teeth or implants where bleeding is anticipated; (2) respiratory tract procedures including tonsillectomy and adenoidectomy, surgical operations involving the respiratory mucosa, and bronchoscopy with a rigid bronchoscope; and (3) genitourinary tract procedures including prostatic surgery, cystoscopy, and urethral dilation.

[e]Prophylaxis for high-risk but not moderate-risk patients is recommended for patients undergoing gastrointestinal tract procedures including sclerotherapy, esophageal stricture dilation, ERCP with biliary obstruction, biliary tract surgery, surgical operations involving the intestinal mucosa, and colon and rectal endoscopy. (Dis Colon Rectum 2000;43:1193)

FALLS IN THE ELDERLY

Older person who:
- Presents for medical attention due to a fall, or
- Reports ≥ 1 fall in past year, or
- Demonstrates abnormalities of gait and/or balance

↓

Fall evaluation:
- History: fall circumstances, medications, acute or chronic medical problems, mobility
- Exam: vision, gait and balance, lower extremity joint function, neurologic function (mental status; muscle strength; lower extremity peripheral nerves; proprioception; reflexes; cortical, extrapyramidal, and cerebellar function), cardiovascular status (heart rate and rhythm, postural pulse and blood pressure, heart rate and blood pressure response to carotid sinus stimulation)

↓

Multifactorial interventions:
(as appropriate, based on evaluation)
- Appropriate use of assistive devices
- Exercise programs, with balance training
- Gait training
- Modification of environmental hazards
- Review and modification of medications, especially psychotropics
- Staff education at long-term care and assisted-living settings
- Treatment of cardiovascular disorders
- Treatment of postural hypotension

Source: JAGS 2001;49:664–672 and NEJM 2003;348:42–49.

	HYPERTENSION	
Disease Prevention		
Organization		
Date		
Population		
Recommendations		
Comments		
Source		

Disease Prevention	Organization	Date	Population	Recommendations	Comments	Source
Hypertension	JNC VII NHLBI	2003 2003	Persons at risk for developing hypertension[a]	Recommend weight loss, reduced sodium intake, moderate alcohol consumption, increased physical activity, potassium supplementation, modification of eating patterns[b]	1. A 5-mm Hg reduction of SBP in the population would result in a 14% overall reduction in mortality due to stroke, a 9% reduction in mortality due to coronary heart disease, and a 7% decrease in all-cause mortality. 2. Weight loss of as little as 10 lb (4.5 kg) reduces BP and/or prevents hypertension in a large proportion of overweight patients.	Hypertension 2003;42:1206–1252

[a]Family history of hypertension; African-American (black race) ancestry; overweight or obesity; sedentary lifestyle; excess intake of dietary sodium; insufficient intake of fruits, vegetables, and potassium; excess consumption of alcohol.
[b]See Lifestyle Modifications for Primary Prevention of Hypertension on page 72.

LIFESTYLE MODIFICATIONS FOR PRIMARY PREVENTION OF HYPERTENSION

- Maintain normal body weight for adults (BMI, 18.5–24.9 kg/m^2)
- Reduce dietary sodium intake to no more than 100 mmol/day (approximately 6 g of sodium chloride or 2.4 g of sodium/day)
- Engage in regular aerobic physical activity such as brisk walking (at least 30 minutes/day, most days of the week)
- Limit alcohol consumption to no more than 2 drinks [e.g., 24 oz (720 mL) of beer, 10 oz (300 mL) of wine, or 3 oz (90 mL) of 100-proof whiskey] per day in most men and to no more than 1 drink per day in women and lighter-weight persons
- Maintain adequate intake of dietary potassium [> 90 mmol (3,500 mg)/day]
- Consume a diet that is rich in fruits and vegetables and in low-fat dairy products with a reduced content of saturated and total fat [Dietary Approaches to Stop Hypertension (DASH) eating plan]

MYOCARDIAL INFARCTION					
Disease Prevention	Organization	Date	Population	Recommendations	Comments	Source
Myocardial Infarction	USPSTF	2004	Adults at low risk of CHD events	Recommend against routine screening with resting electrocardiography (ECG), exercise-treadmill test (ETT), or electron-beam CT (EBCT).	1. Based on the Nurses' Health Study, women adhering to all 4 recommendations had a relative risk of coronary events of 0.17 compared to all other women. (NEJM 2000;343:16)	Ann Intern Med 2004;140:569–572
	USPSTF	2004	Adults at increased risk of CHD events	Insufficient evidence to recommend for or against routine screening with ECT, ETT, or EBCT.		Ann Intern Med 2004;140:569–572
	AHA	2002	All	Begin risk factor assessment at age 20 years. *Dietary guidelines:* (1) Match energy intake with energy needs. (2) Reduce saturated fat (< 10% calories), cholesterol (< 300 mg/day), and trans-fatty acids by substituting grains and unsaturated fatty acids. (3) Limit salt intake (< 6 g/day). (4) Limit alcohol (≤ 2 drinks/day in men; ≤ 1 drink per day in women). *Physical activity:* ≥ 30 minutes of moderate intensity (15–20 minutes/mile) for most days of week. *Control weight:* Achieve and maintain BMI at 18.5–24.9 kg/m^2 (see Appendix IV: BMI Conversion Table). Strongly encourage *smoking cessation.*		Circulation 2002;106:388 Circulation 2000;102:2284

	MYOCARDIAL INFARCTION				
Disease Prevention	**Organization**	**Date**	**Population**	**Recommendations**	**Comments**	**Source**
Myocardial Infarction (continued)	AHA NCEP III	2002 2002	Hyperlipidemia[a]	For screening recommendations, see page 31; also see NCEP III screening and management (page 108) recommendations.	1. Short-term reduction in LDL using dietary counseling by dietitians is superior to that achieved by physicians. (Am J Med 2000;109:549)	Circulation 2002;106:338 Circulation 2004;110:227–239
	JNC VII	2003	Hypertension	See page 117 for JNC VII treatment algorithms.	1. Meta-analysis suggests that beta-blockers should not be first-line therapy for uncomplicated hypertension in persons aged > 60 years. (JAMA 1998;279:1903)	Hypertension 2003;42:1206–1252
	AHA	2002	Hypertension	Goal: < 140/90; < 130/85 if renal insufficiency or heart failure present; < 130/80 if diabetes present.	2. Antiplatelet therapy with ASA not recommended for primary prevention (benefit negated by harm). Antiplatelet therapy recommended for secondary prevention. Lack of demonstrated benefit of warfarin therapy. Glycoprotein IIb/IIIa inhibitors, ticlopidine, and clopidogrel have not been sufficiently evaluated in patients with hypertension. (Cochrane Database Syst Rev 2004;3:CD003186)	Circulation 2002;106:388

MYOCARDIAL INFARCTION

Disease Prevention	Organization	Date	Population	Recommendations	Comments	Source
Myocardial Infarction (continued)	ACP	2004	Diabetes	Statins should be used for primary prevention against macrovascular complications if have type 2 DM and other cardiovascular risk factors (age > 55 years, left ventricular hypertrophy, previous cerebrovascular disease, peripheral arterial disease).		Ann Intern Med 2004;140:644–649
	AHA	2002	Diabetes	Goals: normal fasting glucose (< 110 mg/dL) and near normal HbA1c (< 7%).	1. ACE inhibitors should be first choice for diabetics with hypertension (NEJM 1998;338:645, BMJ 1998;317:703, Diabetes Care 1998;21:597), and may be superior in reducing risk for acute MI, but not stroke. (Diabetes Care 2000;23:888, J Hypertens 2000;18:1671) 2. Studies are supporting more aggressive BP control in this population (eg, < 130/80 mm Hg). (Lancet 1998;351:1755)	Circulation 2002;106:388

Disease Prevention	Organization	Date	Population	Recommendations	Comments	Source
Myocardial Infarction (continued)	AHA	2004	Women	Smoking cessation. Physical activity. Heart-healthy diet. BMI 18.5–24.9 kg/m². Waist circumference <35 in. Evaluate and treat for depression. Omega-3-fatty acids and folic acid if high risk.[b] BP < 120/80. Lipids: LDL-C < 100 mg/dL, HDL-C > 50 mg/dL, triglycerides < 150 mg/dL. Aspirin (75–162 mg) or clopidogrel if high risk[b] (not recommended if low risk). Beta-blockers if history of myocardial infarction or chronic ischemic syndromes. ACE inhibitors if high risk.[b] Estrogen plus progestin hormone therapy should NOT be used or continued. Antioxidant supplements NOT recommended.		Circulation 2004;109:672–693

[a]RCTs have demonstrated the CHD and mortality benefit and safety of treatment of patients with hypercholesterolemia (pravastatin, 40 mg/day) (NEJM 1995;333:1301) and the CHD benefit of treatment of average cholesterol and LDL levels (but low HDL) (lovastatin, 20–40 mg/day). (JAMA 1998;279:1615)

[b]High risk: CHD or risk equivalent or 10-year absolute CHD risk >20%.

OSTEOPOROSIS

Disease Prevention	Organization	Date	Population	Recommendations	Comments	Source
Osteoporosis	ACOG AAFP NOF AACE NIH	2003 2002 2002 2001 2001	Women	Counsel all women about fracture risk reduction (dietary calcium, vitamin D, weight-bearing exercise, smoking cessation, moderate alcohol intake).[a] ACOG continues to support the judicious, individualized use of estrogen and progestin for bone protection. *Alendronate:* Approved for prevention of bone loss in recently menopausal women and treatment of established osteoporosis in men and women. Has been shown to increase BMD by 5%–10% and to decrease fracture incidence by 50%.[c] *Risedronate:* Approved for prevention and treatment of postmenopausal and glucocorticoid-induced osteoporosis. Has been shown to increase BMD and decrease fracture incidence by 30%–50%.[c] *Raloxifene:* Approved for prevention and treatment of postmenopausal osteoporosis. Has been shown to decrease the risk of vertebral fracture by 50% and to increase BMD.[f]	1. Medical disorders associated with osteoporosis include hypogonadism (men),[b] thyroid hormone excess, hypercalciuria, hyperparathyroidism, and malabsorption. Anticonvulsant therapy and use of glucocorticoids are also associated with osteoporosis. 2. For women receiving thyroid replacement therapy for nonmalignant conditions, periodically monitor TSH levels and adjust dose. 3. Predictors of low bone mass include increased age, estrogen deficiency, white race, low weight and BMI, smoking, history of prior fractures, oral or inhaled glucocorticoid therapy use.[d] Use of alcohol and caffeine-containing beverages is inconsistently associated with decreased bone mass. Grip strength and current exercise are associated with increased bone mass.	http://www.acog.org http://www.aafp.org/ http://www.nof.org JAMA 2001;285:785–795 Endocrine Practice 2001;4:293–312 NEJM 2001;345:941–947; 989–992

OSTEOPOROSIS						
Disease Prevention	**Organization**	**Date**	**Population**	**Recommendations**	**Comments**	**Source**
Osteoporosis (continued)					4. Women's Health Initiative found that use of conjugated equine estrogen (0.625 mg/day) and medroxyprogesterone acetate (2.5 mg/day) reduced the risk of hip fracture by 33%. The change in bone mineral density after 3 years was 4.5% higher for lumbar spine and 3.6% higher for total hip for hormone users vs. non-users. (JAMA 2003;290:1729–1748) 5. Statin use did not improve fracture risk or bone density in the Women's Health Initiative Observational Study. (Ann Intern Med 2003;139:97–104)	

[a]Recommended calcium: 9–18 years, 1,500 mg/day; 19–50 years, 1,000 mg/day; > 50 years, 1,200 mg/day. Recommended vitamin D: 400–800 IU/day.

[b]Early evidence indicates that testosterone replacement therapy may enhance bone mass in hypogonadal men; longer-term studies are needed to better define risks and benefits. (JAGS 2001;49:179–187)

[c]Recommended dose: 5 mg/day (35 mg per week) for recently menopausal women; 10 mg/day (70 mg per week) for established osteoporosis. Treatment efficacy demonstrated for 7 years.

[d]Consider bisphosphonate (alendronate or risedronate) for all adult women who require > 7.5 mg prednisone (or equivalent) for > 3 weeks.

[e]Recommended dose 5 mg/day.

[f]Recommended dosing: 60 mg/day.

OSTEOPOROSIS: PREVENTION FOR WOMEN AT RISK*

1. <u>COUNSEL ON:</u>
   - Tobacco cessation
   - Limit alcohol intake
   - Regular weight-bearing exercise ≥ 30 min. 3x/week
     Muscle strengthening exercise
   - Adequate Ca^{2+} intake 1,000–1,200 mg/day
     Adequate vitamin D 800 IU/day

2. <u>IDENTIFY AND REMEDY
   SECONDARY CAUSES</u>
   (see table, page 55)

PERIMENOPAUSAL/POSTMENOPAUSAL	ELDERLY

- Identify and treat sensory deficits, neurologic disease & arthritis, all of which can lead to ↑ frequency of falls
- Adjust drug dosages for drugs that are sedating, slow reflexes, ↓ coordination & impair a person's ability to break impact of a fall
- Gait & balance training to ↓ risk of falls
- Identify and treat ♀ with osteoporosis-related fractures and those with low bone mass.

- See perimenopausal/ postmenopausal recommendations; in addition:
  - Anchor rugs
  - Minimize clutter
  - Remove loose wires
  - Use non-skid mats
  - Add handrails in halls, bathrooms, & stairwells
  - Ensure adequate lighting in halls, stairwells, & entrances
  - Wear sturdy, low-heeled shoes

Source: Adapted from AACE clinical practice guidelines for the prevention & treatment of postmenopausal osteoporosis.

*See page 54 for description of risks.

STROKE

Disease Prevention	Organization	Date	Population	Recommendations	Comments	Source
Stroke	JNC VII AHA	2003 2002	Hypertension	See Myocardial Infarction (pages 73–76) and Hypertension Management (pages 117–120).		Hypertension 2003;42:1206–1252 Circulation 2002;106:388 Ann Intern Med 2003;139:1009
	AAFP ACP	2003 2003	Atrial fibrillation	See Management algorithm, page 103. Prioritize rate control; de-emphasize rhythm	1. Average stroke rate in patients with risk factors about 5% per year (in those with no Hx of stroke or TIA).	Ann Intern Med 2003;139:1009
	ACCP	2001	Atrial fibrillation	Give anticoagulation with warfarin; target prothrombin time INR = 2.5 (range, 2.0–3.0). All patients with any high risk factor for stroke[b] or > 1 moderate risk factor for stroke[c]: Give warfarin as above. Patients with 1 moderate risk factor[c]: Give aspirin or oral anticoagulants. Patients with no high or moderate risk factors: Give aspirin, 325 mg/day.	2. Meta-analysis concluded that adjusted-dose warfarin reduced the absolute risk of stroke by about 2.7% per year (NNT = 37) compared with 1.5% reduction for aspirin (NNT = 67). Risk of major bleed = 0.6% per year (NNH = 167); risk of intracranial bleed = 0.3% per year (NNH = 333). (Am Intern Med 1999;131:492) 3. For mechanical heart valve recommendations, see Chest 2001;119 (1 Suppl):220S–227S.	Chest 2001;119 (1 Suppl):194S
	AHA	2001	Atrial fibrillation	Goal: anticoagulation with INR 2.0–3.0 (target, 2.5) Aged < 65 years, no risk factors: aspirin Aged < 65 years, w/risk factors[a]: warfarin (INR 2.0–3.0) Aged 65–75 years, no risk factors: aspirin or warfarin Aged 65–75 years w/risk factors: warfarin (INR 2.0–3.0) Aged > 75 years: warfarin (INR 2.0–3.0)		Circulation 2001;104:2118–2150

Disease Prevention	Organization	Date	Population	Recommendations	Comments	Source
Stroke (continued)	AHA	2002	Diabetes	See Myocardial Infarction pages 73–76.		Circulation 2002;106:388
	AHA	2001	Carotid artery stenosis	See Disease Screening: Carotid Artery Stenosis for screening and treatment guidelines. Clear consensus exists on efficacy of treatment for symptomatic CAS; treatment of asymptomatic CAS is controversial.[d]		Circulation 2001;103:163 CMAJ 1997;157:653 J Vasc Surg 1992;15:469
	AHA NCEP III	2002 2002	Hyperlipidemia	See screening recommendations on page 31. See Myocardial Infarction (pages 73–76). See Cholesterol and Lipid Management (pages 108–110). Statin initiation during hospitalization for first ischemic stroke of atherosclerotic origin is probably justified.		Circulation 2002;106:388 JAMA 2001;285:2486 Circulation 2004;110:227–239 Stroke 2002;35:1023
	AHA	2002	Smoking	Strongly encourage patient and family to stop smoking. Provide counseling, nicotine replacement, and formal programs as available.		Circulation 2002;106:388

[a] Atrial fibrillation risk factors: hypertension, diabetes mellitus, poor left ventricular function, rheumatic mitral valve disease, prior TIA/stroke, systemic embolism or stroke, prosthetic heart valve (may require higher target INR).

[b] High risk factors for stroke in patients with atrial fibrillation include previous transient ischemic attack or stroke or embolus, hypertension, poor LV function, age > 75 years, diabetes, rheumatic mitral valve disease, and prosthetic heart valves.

[c] Moderate risk factors for stroke are age 65–75 years, diabetes, and coronary artery disease with preserved LV function.

[d] Net benefit of carotid endarterectomy requires treatment by surgical team with low perioperative risk of stroke/death (< 3%) and is enhanced for patients with symptomatic CAS when performed early (within 2 weeks of last ischemic event). (Lancet 2004;363:915)

RECOMMENDED CHILDHOOD IMMUNIZATION SCHEDULE (ACIP, AAP, AAFP)

Vaccine	Birth	1 mo	2 mo	4 mo	6 mo	12 mo	15 mo	18 mo	24 mo	4–6 y	11–12 y	14–18 y
HBV[b]	Hep B #1	only if mother HBsAg(−)										
		Hep B #2			Hep B #3				Hep B series[c]			
DTaP[d]			DTaP	DTaP	DTaP		DTaP[d]			DTaP	Td[e]	
Hib[e]			Hib	Hib	Hib	Hib						
Inactivated polio virus			IPV	IPV	IPV					IPV		
Pneumococcal conjugate[f]			PCV	PCV	PCV	PCV			PCV[e]		PPV[e]	
MMR[g]						MMR #1				MMR #2	MMR[e] #2	
Varicella[h]						Var				Var[c]		
HAV[i]										Hep A series		
Influenza[j]						FLU[j,k]						

Age[a]

Shading indicates range of acceptable ages for vaccination. Any dose not given at the recommended age should be given as a "catch-up" immunization at any subsequent visit when indicated and feasible.

[a] This schedule indicates the recommended ages for routine administration of currently licensed childhood vaccines, as of 8/1/04. Additional vaccines may be licensed and recommended during the year. Providers should consult the manufacturers' package inserts for detailed recommendations.

[b] *All infants* should receive the first dose of hepatitis B vaccine soon after birth and before hospital discharge; the first dose may be given by age 2 months if the mother is HBs-Ag-negative. Only monovalent hepatitis B vaccine can be used for the birth dose. Monovalent or combination vaccine containing hepatitis B may be used to complete the series. The second dose should be given at least 4 weeks after the first, except for combination vaccines, which cannot be administered before age 6 weeks. The third dose should be administered at least 16 weeks after the first dose and at least 8 weeks after the second dose, but not before age 6 months. *Infants of HBs-Ag-positive mothers* should receive hepatitis B vaccine and 0.5 mL hepatitis B immune globulin (HBIG) within 12 hours of birth at separate sites. The second dose is recommended at 1–2 months of age, and the third dose at age 6 months. These infants should be tested for HBs-Ag and anti-HBs at 9–15 months of age. *Infants for whom maternal HBs-Ag status is unknown* should receive hepatitis B vaccine within 12 hours of birth. Maternal blood should be drawn as soon as possible to determine maternal HBsAg status; if the HBs-Ag is positive, the infant should receive hepatitis B immune globulin as soon as possible (no later than age 1 week). The second dose is recommended at 1–2 months of age, and the third dose at age 6 months. All children and adolescents (through age 18 years) who have not been vaccinated against hepatitis B may begin the series during any visit. Special efforts should be made to vaccinate children who were born in or whose parents were born in areas of the world where HBV infection is moderately or highly endemic.

[c] Vaccines to be assessed and administered if necessary.

[d] Td (tetanus and diphtheria toxoids) is recommended at age 11–12 years if at least 5 years have elapsed since the last dose of DTP, DTaP, or DT. Subsequent routine Td boosters are recommended every 10 years.

[e] Three *Haemophilus influenzae* type b (Hib) conjugate vaccines are licensed for infant use. If PRP-OMP (PedvaxHIB® or ComVax®) is administered at ages 2 and 4 months, a dose at age 6 months is not required. DTaP/Hib combination products should not be used for primary immunization in infants at 2, 4, or 6 months of age, but can be used for boosters following any Hib vaccine.

[f] The heptavalent conjugate pneumococcal vaccine (PCV) is recommended for all children 2–23 months of age. It also is recommended for certain children 24–59 months of age. Pneumococcal polysaccharide vaccine (PPV) is recommended in addition to PCV for certain high-risk groups (chronic cardiac or pulmonary disease, diabetes mellitus, anatomic asplenia, chronic renal failure, nephrotic syndrome, sickle cell disease, acquired or congenital immunodeficiency).

gThe second dose of MMR is recommended routinely at age 4–6 years but may be administered during any visit, provided at least 4 weeks have elapsed since receipt of the first dose and that both doses are administered beginning at or after age 12 months. Those who have not previously received the second dose should complete the schedule no later than the routine visit at age 11–12 years.

hVaricella vaccine is recommended at any visit on or after age 12 months for susceptible children (ie, those who lack a reliable history of chickenpox and who have not been vaccinated). Susceptible persons aged ≥ 13 years should receive 2 doses given at least 4 weeks apart.

iHepatitis A vaccine is recommended for children and adolescents in selected states and regions and for certain high-risk groups; consult your local public health authority. Children and adolescents in these states, regions, and high-risk groups who have not been immunized against hepatitis A can begin the series during any visit. The 2 doses in the series should be administered ≥ 6 months apart.

jInactivated influenza vaccine is preferred over live, attenuated vaccine (LAIV) for vaccinating household members, health care workers, and others in close contact with severely immunosuppressed persons during periods when such persons require care in a protected environment. If a health care worker receives LAIV, he or she should refrain from contact with severely immunosuppressed persons for 7 days.

kBecause of unanticipated shortages of influenza vaccine in 2004/2005, the CDC strongly recommends that influenza vaccine be prioritized for all children aged 6–23 months and children aged 2–17 years with underlying chronic medical conditions or receiving chronic aspirin therapy. Intranasally administered, live, attenuated influenza vaccine, if available, should be encouraged for healthy persons who are aged 5–49 years and are not pregnant. Certain children aged < 9 years require 2 doses of vaccine if they have not previously been vaccinated. All children at high risk for complications from influenza, including those aged 6–23 months, who present for vaccination should be vaccinated with a first or second dose, depending on vaccination status. However, doses should not be held in reserve to ensure that 2 doses will be available. Instead, available vaccine should be used to vaccinate persons in priority groups on a first-come, first-served basis.

Source: http://www.cdc.gov/nip

Recommended Adult Immunization Schedule, United States, 2003–2004

by Age Group

Vaccine ▼ Age Group ▶	19–49 Years	50–64 Years	65 Years and Older
Tetanus, diphtheria (Td)*	1 dose booster every 10 years[1]		
Influenza	1 dose annually[2]		1 dose annually[2]
Pneumococcal (polysaccharide)	1 dose[3,4]		1 dose[3,4]
Hepatitis B*	3 doses (0, 1–2, 4–6 months)[5]		
Hepatitis A	2 doses (0, 6–12 months)[6]		
Measles, Mumps, Rubella (MMR)*	1 dose if measles, mumps, or rubella vaccination history is unreliable; 2 doses for persons with occupational or other indications[7]		
Varicella*	2 doses (0, 4–8 weeks) for persons who are susceptible[8]		
Meningococcal (polysaccharide)	1 dose[9]		

Legend: ■ For all persons in this group ▨ Catch-up on childhood vaccinations ▨ For persons with medical/exposure indications ■ Contraindicated

*Covered by the Vaccine Injury Compensation Program. For information on how to file a claim, call 800-338-2382. Please also visit http://www.hrsa.gov/osp/vicp. To file a claim for vaccine injury, write: U.S. Court of Federal Claims, 717 Madison Place, N.W., Washington D.C. 20005. 202-219-9657.

This schedule indicates the recommended age groups for routine administration of currently licensed vaccines for persons 19 years of age and older. Licensed combination vaccines may be used whenever any components of the combination are indicated and the vaccine's other components are not contraindicated. Providers should consult the manufacturers' package inserts for detailed recommendations.

Report all clinically significant post-vaccination reactions to the Vaccine Adverse Event Reporting System (VAERS). Reporting forms and instructions on filing a VAERS report are available by calling 800-822-7967 or from the VAERS website at http://www.vaers.org.

For additional information about the vaccines listed above and contraindications for immunization, visit the National Immunization Program website at http://www.cdc.gov/nip/ or call the National Immunization Hotline at 800-232-2522 (English) or 800-232-0233 (Spanish).

Recommended Adult Immunization Schedule, United States, 2003–2004

Vaccine / Medical Conditions — by Medical Conditions

Medical Conditions ▼ / Vaccine ▶	Tetanus-diphtheria (Td)*,1	Influenza2	Pneumococcal (polysaccharide)3,4	Hepatitis B*,5	Hepatitis A6	Measles, Mumps, Rubella (MMR)*,7	Varicella*,8
Pregnancy		A					
Diabetes, heart disease, chronic pulmonary disease, chronic liver disease, including chronic alcoholism		B	C	D			F
Congenital immunodeficiency, leukemia, lymphoma, generalized malignancy, therapy with alkylating agents, antimetabolites, radiation, or large amounts of corticosteroids			E				
Renal failure/end stage renal disease, recipients of hemodialysis or clotting factor concentrates			E	G			
Asplenia including elective splenectomy and terminal complement component deficiencies			E, I, J				
HIV infection		H	E, H			L	

Legend:
- ▓ For all persons in this group
- ▒ Catch-up on childhood vaccinations
- ▒ (gray) For persons with medical/exposure indications
- ■ Contraindicated

Special Notes for Medical Conditions

A. For women without chronic diseases/conditions, vaccinate if pregnancy will be at 2nd or 3rd trimester during influenza season. For women with chronic diseases/conditions, vaccinate at any time during the pregnancy.

B. Although chronic liver disease and alcoholism are not indicator conditions for influenza vaccination, give 1 dose annually if the patient is ≥ 50 years, has other indicators for influenza vaccine, or if the patient requests vaccination.

C. Asthma is an indicator condition for influenza but not for pneumococcal vaccination.

D. For all persons with chronic liver disease.

E. Revaccinate once after 5 years or more have elapsed since initial vaccination or if initial vaccination prior to age 65 years.

F. Persons with impaired humoral but not cellular immunity may be vaccinated. MMWR 1999;48 (RR-06):1–5.

G. Hemodialysis patients: use special formulation of vaccine (40 μg/mL) or two 1.0 mL 20 μg doses given at one site. Vaccinate early in the course of renal disease. Assess antibody titers to hep B surface antigen (anti-HBs) levels annually. Administer additional doses if anti-HBs levels decline to < 10 milliinternational units (mIU)/mL.

H. There are no data specifically on risk of severe or complicated influenza infections among persons with asplenia. However, influenza is a risk factor for secondary bacterial infections that may cause severe disease in asplenics.

I. Administer meningococcal vaccine and consider Hib vaccine.

J. Elective splenectomy: vaccinate at least 2 weeks before surgery.

K. Vaccinate as close to diagnosis as possible when CD4 cell counts are highest.

L. Withhold MMR or other measles-containing vaccines from HIV-infected persons with evidence of severe immunosuppression. MMWR 1998;47 (RR-8):21–22; MMWR 2002;51 (RR-02):22–24.

1. Tetanus and diphtheria (Td)— Adults, including pregnant women with uncertain histories of a complete primary vaccination series, should receive a primary series of Td. A primary series for adults is 3 doses: the first 2 doses given at least 4 weeks apart and the 3rd dose, 6–12 months after the second. Administer 1 dose if the person had received the primary series and the last vaccination was 10 years ago or longer. Consult MMWR 1991;40 (RR-10):1–21 for administering Td as prophylaxis in wound management. The ACP Task Force on Adult Immunization supports a second opinion for Td use in adults: a single Td booster at age 50 years for persons who have completed the full pediatric series, including the teenage/young adult booster. (*Guide for Adult Immunization.* 3rd ed. ACP 1994;20)

2. Influenza vaccination—Medical indications: chronic disorders of the cardiovascular or pulmonary systems including asthma; chronic metabolic diseases including diabetes mellitus, renal dysfunction, hemoglobinopathies, or immunosuppression [including immunosuppression caused by medications or by human immunodeficiency virus (HIV)], requiring regular medical follow-up or hospitalization during the preceding year; women who will be in the second or third trimester of pregnancy during the influenza season. Occupational indications: health care workers. Other indications: residents of nursing homes and other long-term care facilities; persons likely to transmit influenza to persons at high risk (in-home caregivers to persons with medical indications, household contacts and out-of-home caregivers of children birth to 23 months of age, or children with asthma or other indicator conditions for influenza vaccination, household members and caregivers of elderly and adults with high-risk conditions); and anyone who wishes to be vaccinated. For healthy persons aged 5–49 years without high-risk conditions, either the inactivated vaccine or the intranasally administered influenza vaccine (Flumist) may be given. [MMWR 2003;52 (RR-8):1-36; MMWR 2003;52 (RR-13):12]

   UPDATE 2004/2005: Because of unanticipated shortages of influenza vaccine in 2004/2005, the CDC strongly recommends that influenza vaccine be prioritized for all adults aged 65 years and older, adults aged 18–64 years with underlying chronic medical conditions, residents of nursing homes and long-term care facilities, health care workers involved in direct patient care, and out-of-home caregivers and household contacts of children aged < 6 months. Intranasally administered, live, attenuated influenza vaccine, if available, should be encouraged for healthy persons who are aged 5–49 years and are not pregnant.

3. Pneumococcal polysaccharide vaccination—Medical indications: chronic disorders of the pulmonary system (excluding asthma), cardiovascular diseases, diabetes mellitus, chronic liver diseases including liver disease as a result of alcohol abuse (eg, cirrhosis), chronic renal failure or nephrotic syndrome, functional or anatomic asplenia (eg, sickle cell disease or splenectomy), immunosuppressive conditions (eg, congenital immunodeficiency, HIV infection, leukemia, lymphoma, multiple myeloma, Hodgkin's disease, generalized malignancy, organ or bone marrow transplantation), chemotherapy with alkylating agents, anti-metabolites, or long-term systemic corticosteroids. Geographic/other indications: Alaskan Natives and certain American Indian populations. Other indications: residents of nursing homes and other long-term care facilities. [MMWR 1997;47 (RR-8):1–24]

4. Revaccination with pneumococcal polysaccharide vaccine—One-time revaccination after 5 years for persons with chronic renal failure or nephrotic syndrome, functional or anatomic asplenia (eg, sickle cell disease or splenectomy), immunosuppressive conditions (eg, congenital immunodeficiency, HIV infection, leukemia, lymphoma, multiple myeloma, Hodgkin's disease, generalized malignancy, organ or bone marrow transplantation), chemotherapy with alkylating agents, anti-metabolites, or long-term systemic corticosteroids. For persons 65 and older, one-time revaccination if they were vaccinated 5 or more years previously and were aged less than 65 years at the time of primary vaccination. [MMWR 1997;47 (RR-8):1–24]

5. Hepatitis B vaccination—Medical indications: hemodialysis patients, patients who receive clotting-factor concentrates. Occupational indications: health care workers and public-safety workers who have exposure to blood in the workplace, persons in training in schools of medicine, dentistry, nursing, laboratory technology, other allied health professions. Behavioral indications: injecting drug users, persons with more than one sex partner in the previous 6 months, persons with a recently acquired sexually transmitted disease (STD), all clients in STD clinics, men who have sex with men. Other indications: household contacts and sex partners of persons with chronic HBV infection, clients and staff of institutions for the developmentally disabled, international travelers who will be in countries with high or intermediate prevalence of chronic HBV infection for more than 6 months, inmates of correctional facilities. [MMWR 1991;40 (RR-13):1–25; http://www.cdc.gov/travel/diseases/hbv.htm]

6. Hepatitis A vaccination—For the combined HepA-HepB vaccine, use 3 doses at 0, 1, and 6 months. Medical indications: persons with clotting-factor disorders or chronic liver disease. Behavioral indications: men who have sex with men, users of injecting and noninjecting illegal drugs. Occupational indications: persons working with HAV-infected primates or with HAV in a research laboratory setting. Other indications: persons traveling to or working in countries that have high or intermediate endemicity of hepatitis A. [MMWR 1999;48 (RR-12):1–37;http://www.cdc.gov/travel/diseases/hav.htm]

7. Measles, Mumps, Rubella vaccination (MMR)—Measles component: Adults born before 1957 may be considered immune to measles. Adults born in or after 1957 should receive at least one dose of MMR unless they have a medical contraindication, documentation of at least one dose or other acceptable evidence of immunity. A second dose of MMR is recommended for adults who, were recently exposed to measles or in an outbreak setting, were previously vaccinated with killed measles vaccine, were vaccinated with an unknown vaccine between 1963 and 1967, are students in postsecondary educational institutions, work in health care facilities, plan to travel internationally. Mumps component: 1 dose of MMR should be adequate for protection. Rubella component: Give 1 dose of MMR to women whose rubella vaccination history is unreliable and counsel women to avoid becoming pregnant for 4 weeks after vaccination. For women of child-bearing age, regardless of birth year, routinely determine rubella immunity and counsel women regarding congenital rubella syndrome. Do not vaccinate pregnant women or those planning to become pregnant in the next 4 weeks. If pregnant and susceptible, vaccinate as early in postpartum period as possible. [MMWR 1998;47 (RR-8):1–57; MMWR 2001;50:1117]

8. Varicella vaccination—Recommended for all persons who do not have reliable clinical history of varicella infection, or serological evidence of varicella zoster virus (VZV) infection who may be at high risk for exposure or transmission. This includes health care workers and family contacts of immunosuppressed patients, those who live or work in environments where transmission is likely (eg, teachers of young children, day care employees, and residents and staff members in institutional settings), persons who live or work in environments where VZV transmission can occur (eg, college students, inmates and staff members of correctional institutions, and military personnel), adolescents and adults living in households with children, women who are not pregnant but who may become pregnant in the future, international travelers who are not immune to infection. Note: Greater than 95% of U.S.-born adults are immune to VZV. Do not vaccinate pregnant women or those planning to become pregnant in the next 4 weeks. If pregnant and susceptible, vaccinate as early in the postpartum period as possible. [MMWR 1996;45 (RR-11):1–36; MMWR 1999;48 (RR-6):1–5]

9. Meningococcal vaccine (quadrivalent polysaccharide for serogroups A, C, Y, and W-135)—Consider vaccination for persons with medical indications: adults with terminal complement component deficiencies, with anatomic or functional asplenia. Other indications: travelers to countries in which disease is hyperendemic or epidemic ("meningitis belt" of sub-Saharan Africa; Mecca, Saudi Arabia for Hajj). Revaccination at 3–5 years may be indicated for persons at high risk for infection (eg, persons residing in areas in which disease is epidemic). Counsel college freshmen, especially those who live in dormitories, regarding meningococcal disease and the vaccine so that they can make an educated decision about receiving the vaccination. [MMWR 2000;49:(RR-7):1–20] Note: The AAFP recommends that colleges should take the lead on providing education on meningococcal infection and vaccination and offer it to those who are interested. Physicians need not initiate discussion of the meningococcal quadrivalent polysaccharide vaccine as part of routine medical care.

Recommendations for using smallpox vaccine in a pre-event vaccination program: Smallpox vaccination is recommended for persons designated by public health authorities to conduct investigations and follow-up of initial smallpox cases that might necessitate direct patient contact. ACIP recommends that each state and territory establish and maintain ≥ 1 smallpox response team. Pre-event vaccination is contraindicated for persons with a history or presence of eczema or atopic dermatitis; who have other acute, chronic, or exfoliative skin conditions; who have conditions associated with immunosuppression; who are aged < 1 year; who have a serious allergy to any component of the vaccine; or who are pregnant or breast-feeding, and their household contacts. ACIP does not recommend pre-event vaccination for children and adolescents aged < 18 years. [MMWR 2003;52 (RR-7):1–16]

Source: http://www.cdc.gov/nip

3
Disease Management

ADULT PATIENT WITH ALLERGIC RHINITIS: DIAGNOSIS AND MANAGEMENT
Source: American Academy of Allergy, Asthma and Immunology (AAAAI) and
American College of Allergy, Asthma and Immunology (ACAAI)

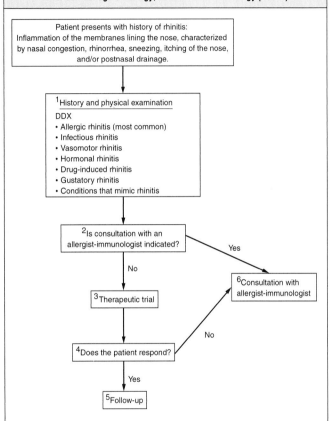

Patient presents with history of rhinitis:
Inflammation of the membranes lining the nose, characterized
by nasal congestion, rhinorrhea, sneezing, itching of the nose,
and/or postnasal drainage.

¹History and physical examination

DDX
• Allergic rhinitis (most common)
• Infectious rhinitis
• Vasomotor rhinitis
• Hormonal rhinitis
• Drug-induced rhinitis
• Gustatory rhinitis
• Conditions that mimic rhinitis

²Is consultation with an
allergist-immunologist indicated?

Yes

No

³Therapeutic trial

⁶Consultation with
allergist-immunologist

⁴Does the patient respond?

No

Yes

⁵Follow-up

Source: Adapted from Diagnosis and Management of Rhinitis: Parameter Documents
of the Joint Task Force on Practice Parameters in Allergy, Asthma and Immunology.
American Academy of Allergy, Asthma and Immunology (AAAAI) and American College
of Allergy, Asthma and Immunology (ACAAI). 1998. (http://www.jcaai.org)

Notes:

1. *History:* (a) presenting symptoms (eg, rhinorrhea, nasal congestion, sneezing, ocular Sx); (b) length of symptomatology; (c) past medications taken for rhinitis, their effectiveness and adverse effects; (d) other medications; (e) degree to which rhinitis Sx interfere with patient's ability to function and affect patient's quality of life; (f) seasonality and known triggers; (g) other medical conditions; (h) complications (eg, otitis media); (i) associated comorbid conditions (eg, asthma). *Physical exam:* (a) evaluation of nose—appearance of nasal mucous membranes, patency of nasal passageways, quality and quantity of nasal discharge; (b) evaluation of ears, eyes, throat, and lungs.

2. Consider initial referral if: (a) need to define allergic/environmental triggers of rhinitis Sx; (b) need for more intense education; (c) requires multiple medications over a prolonged period of time.

3. (a) **Avoidance of inciting factors.**

   (b) **Oral antihistamines:** Effective in reducing symptoms of itching, sneezing, and rhinorrhea. First-line therapy for treatment of allergic rhinitis. Little objective effect on nasal congestion. Second-generation antihistamines that are associated with less risk or no risk for sedation and performance impairment should usually be considered before sedating antihistamines.

   (c) **Intranasal antihistamines:** Appropriate first-line treatment. May help reduce nasal congestion. Sedation may occur from systemic absorption.

   (d) **Oral decongestants:** Can effectively reduce nasal congestion. Can cause insomnia, anorexia, excessive nervousness. May increase BP.

   (e) **Nasally inhaled steroids:** Most effective medication class for controlling Sx of allergic rhinitis. May be considered for initial Tx without a prior trial of antihistamines and/or oral decongestants, and should be considered before initiating Tx with systemic corticosteroids.

   (f) **Oral corticosteroids:** Should be reserved for severe cases of rhinitis. Short burst (5–7 days) preferred over depot parenteral corticosteroids, which should be avoided.

   (g) **Intranasal cromolyn sodium:** Can reduce Sx of allergic rhinitis in some patients; is most likely effective if initiated before Sx become severe.

   (h) **Intranasal anticholinergics:** May effectively reduce rhinorrhea but have no effect on other nasal Sx.

4. Reasons for referral: (a) duration of rhinitis Sx > 3 months; (b) complications of rhinitis (eg, otitis media, sinusitis, nasal polyps); (c) comorbid conditions (eg, asthma); (d) requires oral corticosteroids for rhinitis; (e) symptoms interfere with patient's ability to function; (f) symptoms significantly decrease patient's quality of life; (g) treatment with medications for rhinitis are ineffective or produce adverse events; (h) need to define allergic/environmental triggers of rhinitis Sx; (i) need for more intense education; (j) requires multiple medications over a prolonged period of time.

5. If initial Tx successful, follow patient to assure continued control of Sx, maintenance of improved quality of life, absence of medication side effects, and reinforce education.

6. Additional examination may include: rhinoscopy, immediate hypersensitivity skin tests, or *in vitro* tests to confirm an underlying allergic basis for symptoms. Neither total serum IgE nor total circulating eosinophil counts are routinely indicated as they are neither sensitive nor specific for allergic rhinitis. Specific tests may be necessary for co-existing conditions (eg, asthma, nasal polyps, sinusitis). Specific immunotherapy may be beneficial.

Source: American Academy of Otolaryngic Allergy (AAOA). Allergic rhinitis: clinical practice guideline. Otolaryngol Head Neck Surg 1996;115(1):115–122.

PHARMACOLOGICAL MANAGEMENT OF ARTHRITIS OF HIP AND KNEE
Source: American College of Rheumatology and AAOS

Step-1

Non-Pharmacologic Therapy

- Patient education
- Self-management programs
- Personalized social support through telephone contact
- Weight loss (if overweight)
- Aerobic exercise programs
- Physical therapy
  - Range-of-motion
  - Muscle-strengthening[1]

- Assistive devices for ambulation
- Patellar taping
- Appropriate footwear
- Lateral-wedged insoles (for genu varum)
- Occupational therapy
  - Joint protection
  - Activities of daily living

inadequate symptom relief

Step-2

Acetaminophen[2] (total daily dose not to exceed 4.0 gm/day)
*If moderate-to-severe **inflammation present**, consider **NSAID first.**[3]*

inadequate symptom relief

Step-3

Evaluate Renal and Gastrointestinal Risk

Treatment Options

Renal Risk Present?
creatinine ≥ 2.0 mg/dL
+
(1 of the following)
age ≥ 65 yrs, hypertension,
congestive heart failure, OR
diuretic or ACE inhibitor therapy

Yes →

Non-NSAID Oral Therapy
- *Tramadol*
- *Salsalate*

No ↓

GI Risk Present?
(at least 1 of the following)
age ≥ 65 yrs
comorbidity
oral glucocorticoid Rx
peptic ulcer disease Hx
upper GI bleed Hx
anticoagulant Rx

Yes →

Intraarticular therapy
- *Glucocorticoids*
- *Hyaluronan*[4]
Topical therapy[5]
- *Capsaicin*
- *Methylsalicylate*

Oral Therapy
- *Salsalate*
- *COX-2 inhibitors*[6]
- *NSAID + misoprostol or proton pump inhibitor*
- *Tramadol*

No ↓

Oral Therapy
- *Non-selective NSAID, or other therapies above*[7]

inadequate symptom relief

Step-4

Consider additional or alternative therapies
- **Opioid therapy**
- **Total joint arthroplasty**[8]

Source: Adapted from American College of Rheumatology Subcommittee on Osteoarthritis Guidelines. Recommendations for the Medical Management of Osteoarthritis of the Hip and Knee. Arthritis and Rheumatism 2000;43:1905–1915.

Similar management algorithm offered by AAOS—adds recommendations for radiographs and for knee aspiration (www.aaos.org).

Notes:

1. Quadriceps weakness may precede, initiate, and exacerbate knee osteoarthritis. (Rheum Dis Clin North Am 1999;25:283–398)

2. For many patients with mild to moderate osteoarthritis, pain relief with acetaminophen is comparable to NSAID. (Semin Arthritis Rheum 1997;27:755–770)

3. NSAIDs appear to be superior to acetaminophen in patients with severe pain related to osteoarthritis. (Arthritis Rheum 2000;43:378–385, J Rheumatol 2000;27:1020–1027)

4. Hyaluronan intraarticular therapy has only been evaluated in knee osteoarthritis.

5. Topical therapy primarily indicated for mild to moderate pain related to osteoarthritis of the knee. There are no studies of topical therapy for hip osteoarthritis.

6. COX-2 inhibitors are as efficacious as non-selective NSAIDs, but not more efficacious. In contrast to non-selective NSAIDs, COX-2 inhibitors do not impair platelet function or bleeding time. Note: Rofecoxib withdrawn from market, September 2004.

7. Use of concomitant gastroprotective therapy with misoprostol or a proton pump inhibitor is not recommended in the low-risk patient.

8. In a randomized trial, 180 patients with osteoarthritis of the knee were randomly assigned to receive arthroscopic debridement, arthroscopic lavage, or placebo surgery. The outcomes (pain, physical function) after arthroscopic debridement or lavage were no better than those after the placebo procedure over 24 months of follow-up. (NEJM 2002;347:81–88) However, total joint arthroplasty provides marked pain relief and functional improvement in the vast majority of patients with osteoarthritis, and has been shown to be cost-effective in selected patients. An NIH Consensus conference recommends total hip replacement when "radiographic evidence of joint damage and moderate-to-severe persistent pain and disability, or both, that is not substantially relieved by an extended course of non-surgical management" is present.

EXERCISE PRESCRIPTION FOR OLDER ADULTS WITH OSTEOARTHRITIS PAIN
Source: AGS

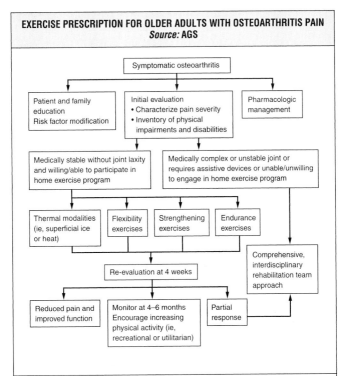

Major risk factors for osteoarthritis: obesity, muscle weakness, heavy physical activity, inactivity, trauma, reduced proprioception, poor joint biomechanics, age, female gender, inheritance, congenital (ie, malformations). Adapted from American Geriatrics Society Consensus Practice Recommendations. (JAGS 2001;49:808–823)

STEPWISE APPROACH FOR MANAGING ASTHMA IN ADULTS AND CHILDREN OLDER THAN 5 YEARS OF AGE

ASTHMA: SEVERITY CLASSIFICATION Source: NHLBI			
DETERMINING ASTHMA SEVERITY			
	Clinical Features before Treatment[a]		
	Symptoms[b]	**Nighttime Symptoms**	**Lung Function**
STEP 1 Mild Intermittent	Symptoms ≤ 2 times a week Asymptomatic and normal PEF between exacerbations Exacerbations brief (from a few hours to a few days); intensity may vary	≤ 2 times a month	FEV1 or PEF = 80% predicted PEF variability < 20%
STEP 2 Mild Persistent	Symptoms > 2 times a week but < 1 time a day Exacerbations may affect activity	> 2 times a month	FEV1 or PEF = 80% predicted PEF variability 20%–30%
STEP 3 Moderate Persistent	Daily symptoms Daily use of inhaled short-acting beta$_2$-agonist Exacerbations affect activity Exacerbations = 2 times a week; may last days	> 1 time a week	FEV1 or PEF > 60% – < 80% predicted PEF variability > 30%
STEP 4 Severe Persistent	Continual symptoms Limited physical activity Frequent exacerbations	Frequent	FEV1 or PEF < 60% predicted PEF variability > 30%

[a]The presence of one of the features of severity is sufficient to place a patient in that category. An individual should be assigned to the most severe grade in which any feature occurs. The characteristics noted in this table are general and may overlap because asthma is highly variable. Furthermore, an individual's classification may change over time.
[b]Patients at any level of severity can have mild, moderate, or severe exacerbations. Some patients with intermittent asthma experience severe and life-threatening exacerbations separated by long periods of normal lung function and no symptoms.
Source: National Heart, Lung and Blood Institute; NIH. http://www.nhlbi.nih.gov/guidelines/asthma/index.htm

ASTHMA: TREATMENT
Source: NHLBI

STEPWISE APPROACH FOR MANAGING ASTHMA IN ADULTS AND CHILDREN OLDER THAN 5 YEARS OF AGE: TREATMENT

Step Down: Review treatment every 1 to 6 months; a gradual stepwise reduction in treatment may be possible.

Step Up: If control is not maintained, consider step up. First, review patient medication technique, adherence, and environmental control (avoidance of allergens or other factors that contribute to asthma severity).

Medications	Mild Intermittent	Mild Persistent	Moderate Persistent	Severe Persistent
Long-term control				
Inhaled steroids (high dose)				X
Inhaled steroids (medium dose)			X or	
Inhaled steroids (low dose) or cromolyn or nedocromil		X or		
Inhaled steroids (low dose) and long-acting bronchodilator[a]			X or	X
Corticosteroid tablets/syrup[b]				X
Sustained release theophylline		X or		
Zafirlukast or zileuton[c]		X or		
Quick relief				
Short-acting bronchodilator[d]	X	X	X	X

STEPWISE APPROACH FOR MANAGING ASTHMA IN ADULTS AND CHILDREN OLDER THAN 5 YEARS OF AGE: TREATMENT (CONTINUED)

ASTHMA: TREATMENT
Source: NHLBI

Step Down: Review treatment every 1 to 6 months; a gradual stepwise reduction in treatment may be possible.

Step Up: If control is not maintained, consider step up. First, review patient medication technique, adherence, and environmental control (avoidance of allergens or other factors that contribute to asthma severity).

	Mild Intermittent	Mild Persistent	Moderate Persistent	Severe Persistent
Education				
Step 1[e]	X	X	X	X
Step 2[f]		X	X	X
Step 3[f]			X	X
Referral				X

ASTHMA: TREATMENT
Source: **NHLBI**

Note: The stepwise approach presents general guidelines to assist clinical decision making; it is not intended to be a specific prescription. Asthma is highly variable; clinicians should tailor specific medication plans to the needs and circumstances of individual patients.

Gain control as quickly as possible; then decrease treatment to the least medication necessary to maintain control. Gaining control may be accomplished by either starting treatment at the step most appropriate to the initial severity of the condition or starting at a higher level or therapy (eg, a course of systemic corticosteroids or higher dose of inhaled corticosteroids).

A rescue course of systemic corticosteroids may be needed at any time and at any step.

Some patients with intermittent asthma experience severe and life-threatening exacerbations separated by long periods of normal lung function and no symptoms. This may be especially common with exacerbations provoked by respiratory infections. A short course of systemic corticosteroids is recommended.

At each step, patients should control their environment to avoid or control factors that make their asthma worse (eg, allergens, irritants); this requires specific diagnosis and education.

Referral to an asthma specialist for consultation or co-management is recommended if there are difficulties achieving or maintaining control of asthma or if the patient requires step 4 care. Referral may be considered if the patient requires step 3 care.

[a]Include long-acting inhaled beta$_2$-agonist, sustained-release theophylline, or long-acting beta$_2$-agonist tablets.

[b]Make repeat attempts to reduce systemic steroids and maintain control with high-dose inhaled steroids.

[c]Consider for patients >12 years of age, although their position in therapy is not fully established.

[d]As needed for symptoms. Intensity of treatment depends on severity of exacerbation. Use of short-acting inhaled beta$_2$-agonists more than 2 times per week may indicate need to initiate long-term therapy.

[e]Teach basic facts about asthma. Teach inhaler/spacer/holding chamber technique. Discuss roles of medications. Develop self-management plan. Develop action plan for when and how to take rescue actions, especially for patients with a history of severe exacerbations. Discuss appropriate environmental control measures to avoid exposure to known allergens and irritants.

[f]Teach self-monitoring. Refer to group education if available. Review and update self-management plan.

Source: NHLBI; NIH. http://www.nhlbi.nih.gov/guidelines/asthma/index.htm

ATOPIC DERMATITIS: EVALUATION & MANAGEMENT ALGORITHM
Source: American College of Allergy, Asthma and Immunology and AAD

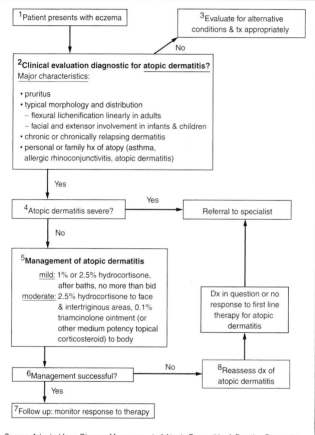

Source: Adapted from Disease Management of Atopic Dermatitis: A Practice Parameter. Am Allergy Asthma Immunol 1997 Sep; 79(3):197–211. (http://www.jcaai.org) and Guidelines of Care for Atopic Dermatitis, AAD, 2003 (www.aad.org).

Notes:

1. **Eczema:** pruritic dermatitis.
2. **Other characteristics of atopic dermatitis** (in the absence of an atopic history, 3 or more required for diagnosis): xerosis; ichthyosis/palmar hyperlinearity/keratosis pilaris; immediate, Type I skin test response; hand and/or foot dermatitis; cheilitis; nipple eczema; susceptibility to cutaneous infections; erythroderma; early age of onset; impaired cell-mediated immunity; recurrent conjunctivitis; infraorbital fold; keratoconus; anterior subscapular cataracts; elevated total serum immunoglobulin E; peripheral blood eosinophils. **History:** pruritic nature of rash, age of onset, duration, triggers, seasonal variation, eye complications, environmental exposures, chronicity, distribution of rash. **Physical examination:** morphology and distribution of the atopic skin lesions, especially diffuse xerosis, erythema, excoriation, papulation, crusting/oozing/pustules indicative of infection, scaling, lichenification. **Laboratory testing:** skin or *in vitro* testing for specific allergens. The majority of patients have elevated serum IgE and eosinophilia; these findings are not useful in guiding clinical decisions. A diagnosis of atopic dermatitis cannot be made solely on the basis of laboratory testing.
3. **Differential diagnosis of atopic dermatitis**
   - *Immunodeficiencies:* Wiskott-Aldrich syndrome, DiGeorge syndrome, Hyper-IgE syndrome, severe combined immune deficiency
   - *Metabolic diseases:* Phenylketonuria, tyrosinemia, histidinemia, multiple carboxylase deficiency, essential fatty acid deficiency
   - *Neoplastic disease:* Cutaneous T-cell lymphoma, histiocytosis X, Sézary syndrome
   - *Infection and infestation:* Candida, herpes simplex, *Staphylococcus aureus, Sarcoptes scabiei*
   - *Dermatitis:* Contact, seborrheic, psoriasis
4. **Severe atopic dermatitis:**
   - More than 20% skin involvement (or 10% skin involvement if affects eyelids, hands, or intertriginous areas)
   - Extensive skin involvement and erythrodermic, at risk for exfoliation
   - Requiring ongoing or frequent treatment with high potency topical glucocorticoids or systemic glucocorticoids
   - Requiring hospitalization for severe eczema or skin infections related to atopic dermatitis
   - Ocular or infectious complications
   - Significant disruption of quality of life
5. Treatment of atopic dermatitis is directed at symptom relief and reduction of cutaneous inflammation. All patients require skin hydration in combination with an effective emollient. Potential trigger factors should be identified and eliminated. Calcineurin inhibitors, pimecrolimus, and tacrolimus have been shown to reduce the extent, severity, and symptoms. Tar may be associated with therapeutic benefits, but is limited by compliance. Short-term adjunctive use of topical doxepin may aid in the reduction of pruritus, but side effects may limit usefulness. Patients with atopic dermatitis are commonly colonized with *Staphylococcus aureus*. Without signs of infection, oral antibiotics have minimal therapeutic effect on the dermatitis. Topical or oral antibiotics can be beneficial when infection is present; development of resistance is a concern.
6. Response to therapy is classified as complete response, partial response, or treatment failure. Most patients will have a partial response with reduction in pruritus and extent of skin disease.
7. Monitor response to therapy and adjust medications and skin care according to severity of illness. Establish a plan to step up medications for flare-ups and to step down medications when the illness is under control.
8. In any patient who fails to respond to treatment, reassess the diagnosis. If presenting after the age of 16 years, consider contact dermatitis. If presenting as an adult, consider cutaneous T-cell lymphoma.

ATRIAL FIBRILLATION: EVALUATION & MANAGEMENT
Source: American Heart Association/American College of Cardiology/European Society of Cardiology

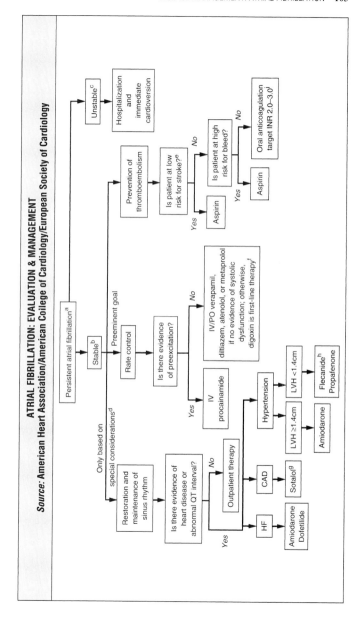

ATRIAL FIBRILLATION: EVALUATION & MANAGEMENT (CONTINUED)
Source: American Heart Association/American College of Cardiology/European Society of Cardiology

[a]Paroxysmal atrial fibrillation episodes last more than 30 seconds, but ≤ 7 days. If ≥ 2 episodes, designate "persistent."

[b]If minimal or no symptoms, anticoagulation, and rate control, "as needed."

[c]Evidence of Wolff-Parkinson-White syndrome of preexcitation, hypotension, or congestive heart failure; ECG evidence of acute MI or symptomatic hypotension, angina, or heart failure.

[d]The AFFIRM trial showed no significant benefit of rhythm control (beyond rate control) in mortality or stroke risk and *increased* risk of death among older patients, those with congestive heart failure, and those with coronary disease. Rhythm control also increased hospitalization and adverse drug effects. (N Engl J Med 2002;347:1825) Special considerations include patient symptoms, exercise tolerance, and patient preference.

[e]Patients at high stroke risk (thromboembolic rates > 5/year) include those with a history of hypertension, prior stroke/transient ischemic attack, diabetes, age > 65 years, impaired systolic function, and enlarged left atrial size. Low-risk patients have a thromboembolic risk of 1.0%–1.5% per year. (Arch Intern Med 1994;154:1449, Ann Intern Med 1992;116:1)

[f]If rate is difficult to control with pharmacologic therapy, consider AV node ablation or modification.

[g]Second-line therapy: amiodarone, dofetilde; third-line: disopyramide, procainamide, quinidine.

[h]Second-line therapy: amiodarone, dofetilide, sotalol; third-line: disopyramide, procainamide, quinidine.

[i]Consider range 1.6 to 2.5 in patients aged > 75 years with increased risk of bleeding complications.

CAD, coronary artery disease; HF, heart failure; LVH, left ventricular hypertrophy.

Source: Adapted from AHA subcommittee on Electrocardiography and Electrophysiology, Circulation 1996;93:1262; and ACC/AHA/ESC, J Am Coll Card 2001;38:1265.

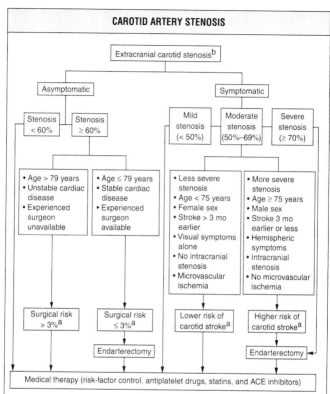

CAROTID ARTERY STENOSIS

Extracranial carotid stenosis[b]

Asymptomatic
- Stenosis < 60%
- Stenosis ≥ 60%

Symptomatic
- Mild stenosis (< 50%)
- Moderate stenosis (50%–69%)
- Severe stenosis (≥ 70%)

Stenosis < 60%:
- Age > 79 years
- Unstable cardiac disease
- Experienced surgeon unavailable

Stenosis ≥ 60%:
- Age ≤ 79 years
- Stable cardiac disease
- Experienced surgeon available

Moderate (less severe):
- Less severe stenosis
- Age < 75 years
- Female sex
- Stroke > 3 mo earlier
- Visual symptoms alone
- No intracranial stenosis
- Microvascular ischemia

Moderate (more severe):
- More severe stenosis
- Age ≥ 75 years
- Male sex
- Stroke 3 mo earlier or less
- Hemispheric symptoms
- Intracranial stenosis
- No microvascular ischemia

- Surgical risk > 3%[a]
- Surgical risk ≤ 3%[a] → Endarterectomy
- Lower risk of carotid stroke[a]
- Higher risk of carotid stroke[a] → Endarterectomy

Medical therapy (risk-factor control, antiplatelet drugs, statins, and ACE inhibitors)

[a]Retrospective review of 1370 CEA (1990–1999) at 1 teaching hospital: no significant difference in incidence of perioperative stroke or death in those with ≥ 1 vs. no risk factors. 30-day mortality significantly greater (2.8% vs. 0.3%, $p = 0.04$) in those with ≥ 2 vs. no risk factors. (J Vasc Surg 2003;37:1191–1199)

[b]Best method for measuring degree of stenosis is angiography.

Source: Adapted from The Guidelines of the American Heart Association and the National Stroke Association. Other factors not included in the figure may also be relevant in risk stratification (eg, the results of cardiac evaluation or hemodynamic testing). Sacco RL. NEJM 2001;345;113.

CATARACT IN ADULTS: EVALUATION & MANAGEMENT ALGORITHM
Source: AHRQ

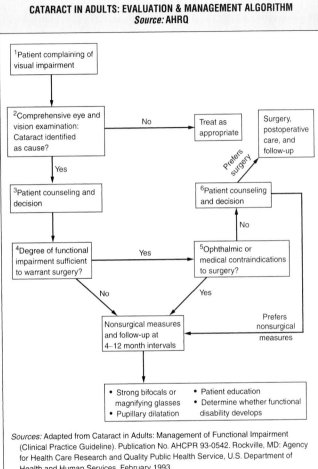

Sources: Adapted from Cataract in Adults: Management of Functional Impairment (Clinical Practice Guideline). Publication No. AHCPR 93-0542. Rockville, MD: Agency for Health Care Research and Quality Public Health Service, U.S. Department of Health and Human Services, February 1993.

American Academy of Ophthalmology and American Society of Cataract and Refractive Surgery. White Paper on Cataract Surgery, 1996.

American Optometric Association Consensus Panel on Care of the Adult Patient with Cataract. Optometric Clinical Practice Guideline: Care of the Adult Patient with Cataract. Updated 3/30/99.

Notes:

1. Begin evaluation only when patients complain of a visual problem or impairment. Identifying impairment in visual function during routine history and physical examination constitutes sound medical practice.

2. Essential elements of the comprehensive eye and vision examination:
   - Patient history. Consider cataract if: acute or gradual onset of vision loss; vision problems under special conditions (eg, low contrast, glare); difficulties performing various visual tasks. Ask about: refractive history, previous ocular disease, amblyopia, eye surgery, trauma, general health history, medications, and allergies. It is critical to describe the actual impact of the cataract on the person's function and quality of life. There are several instruments available for assessing functional impairment related to cataract, including VF-14, Activities of Daily Vision Scale, and Visual Activities Questionnaire.
   - Ocular examination, including: Snellen acuity and refraction; measurement of intraocular pressure; assessment of pupillary function; external examination; slit-lamp examination; and dilated examination of fundus.
   - Supplemental testing: May be necessary to assess and document the extent of the functional disability and to determine whether other diseases may limit preoperative or postoperative vision.
   Most elderly patients presenting with visual problems do not have a cataract that causes functional impairment. Refractive error, macular degeneration, and glaucoma are common alternative etiologies for visual impairment.

3. Once cataract has been identified as the cause of visual disability, patients should be counseled concerning the nature of the problem, its natural history, and the existence of both surgical and nonsurgical approaches to management. The principal factor that should guide decision making with regard to surgery is *the extent to which the cataract impairs the ability to function in daily life.* The findings of the physical examination should corroborate that the cataract is the major contributing cause of the functional impairment, and that there is a reasonable expectation that managing the cataract will positively impact the patient's functional activity. *Visual acuity is not the sole determining factor and should not be used as a threshold value.*

4. Patients who complain of mild to moderate limitation in activities due to a visual problem, those whose corrected acuities are near 20/40, and those who do not yet wish to undergo surgery may be offered nonsurgical measures for improving visual function. Indications for surgery: cataract-impaired vision no longer meets the patient's needs; evidence of lens-induced disease (eg, phakomorphic glaucoma, phakolytic glaucoma); necessary to visualize the fundus in an eye that has the potential for sight (eg, diabetic patient at risk of diabetic retinopathy).

5. *Contraindications to surgery:* the patient does not desire surgery; glasses or visual aids provide satisfactory functional vision; surgery will not improve visual function; the patient's quality of life is not compromised; the patient is unable to undergo surgery because of coexisting medical or ocular conditions; a legal consent cannot be obtained; or the patient is unable to obtain adequate postoperative care. Routine preoperative medical testing (12-lead EKG, CBC, measurement of serum electrolytes, BUN, creatinine, and glucose), while commonly performed in patients scheduled to undergo cataract surgery, does not appear to measurably increase the safety of the surgery.

6. Patients with significant functional and visual impairment due to cataract who have no contraindications to surgery should be counseled regarding the expected risks and benefits of and alternatives to surgery.

CHOLESTEROL & LIPID MANAGEMENT
Source: NCEP III

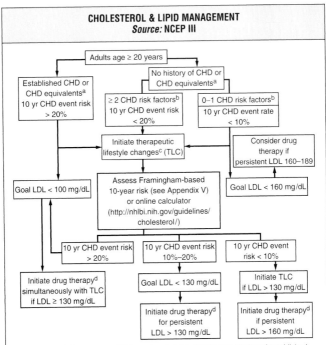

[a]CHD risk equivalents carry a risk for major coronary events equal to that of established CHD (ie, > 20% per 10 years), and include: diabetes, other clinical forms of arthrosclerotic disease (peripheral arterial disease, abdominal aortic aneurysm, and symptomatic carotid artery disease).

[b]Age (men ≥ 45 years, women ≥ 55 years or postmenopausal), hypertension (BP ≥ 140/90 mm Hg or on antihypertensive medication), cigarette smoking, HDL < 40 mg/dL, family history of premature CHD in first-degree relative (males < 55 years, females < 65 years). Diabetes now considered CHD risk equivalent. For HDL ≥ 60 mg/dL, subtract 1 risk factor from above.

[c]All patients, particularly those with elevated cholesterol levels, should be encouraged to adopt the following lifestyle changes: reduce saturated fat (< 7% total calories) and cholesterol (< 200 mg/d intake; increase physical activity; and achieve appropriate weight control (see publication for greater details on TLC regimens). Assess effects of TLC on lipid levels after 3 months.

[d]Drug therapy response should be monitored and modified at 6-week intervals to achieve goal LDL levels; after goal LDL met, monitor response and adherence every 4–6 months.

Source: Executive summary of the third report of the National Cholesterol Education Project (NCEP) expert panel on detection, evaluation and treatment of high blood cholesterol in adults (Adult Treatment Panel III). JAMA 2001;285:2486. Implications of Recent Clinical Trials for the National Cholesterol Education Program Adult Treatment Panel III Guidelines, Circulation 2004;110:227–239.

MODIFICATIONS TO THE
ATP III TREATMENT ALGORITHM FOR LDL-C

In high-risk persons, the recommended LDL-C goal is < 100 mg/dL.

An LDL-C goal of < 70 mg/dL is a therapeutic option, especially for patients at very high risk.

If LDL-C is ≥ 100 mg/dL, an LDL-lowering drug is indicated simultaneously with lifestyle changes.

If baseline LDL-C is < 100 mg/dL, institution of an LDL-lowering drug to achieve an LDL-C level < 70 mg/dL is a therapeutic option.

If a high-risk person has high triglycerides or low HDL-C, consideration can be given to combining a fibrate or nicotinic acid with an LDL-lowering drug. When triglycerides are ≥ 200 mg/dL, non–HDL-C is a secondary target of therapy, with a goal 30 mg/dL higher than the identified LDL-C goal.

For moderately high-risk persons (2+ risk factors and 10-year risk 10%–20%), the recommended LDL-C goal is < 130 mg/dL; an LDL-C goal < 100 mg/dL is a therapeutic option. When LDL-C level is 100–129 mg/dL, at baseline or on lifestyle therapy, initiation of an LDL-lowering drug to achieve an LDL-C level < 100 mg/dL is a therapeutic option.

Any person at high risk or moderately high risk who has lifestyle-related risk factors (e.g., obesity, physical inactivity, elevated triglyceride, low HDL-C, or metabolic syndrome) is a candidate for TLC to modify these risk factors regardless of LDL-C level.

When LDL-lowering drug therapy is employed in high-risk or moderately high-risk persons, intensity of therapy should be sufficient to achieve at least a 30%–40% reduction in LDL-C levels.

Source: Implications of Recent Clinical Trials for the National Cholesterol Education Program Adult Treatment Panel III guidelines. Circulation 2004;110:227–239.

METABOLIC SYNDROME: IDENTIFICATION AND MANAGEMENT

Clinical Identification

Risk Factor	Defining Level
Abdominal obesity (waist circumference)	
Men	≥ 102 cm (≥ 40 in.)
Women	≥ 88 cm (≥ 35 in.)
Triglycerides	≥ 150 mg/dL
HDL cholesterol	
Men	< 40 mg/dL
Women	< 50 mg/dL
Blood pressure	≥ 130/≥ 85 mm Hg
Fasting glucose	≥ 110 mg/dL

Management

First-line therapy: Lifestyle modification leading to weight reduction and increased physical activity.

Goal: ↓ Body weight by ~7%–10% over 6–12 months.

Daily minimum: 30 minutes of moderate-intensity physical activity.

Low intake of saturated fats, trans fats, and cholesterol.

Reduced consumption of simple sugars.

Increased intake of fruits, vegetables, and whole grains.

Avoid extremes in intake of either carbohydrates or fats.

Smoking cessation.

Drug therapy for hypertension, elevated LDL cholesterol, and diabetes.

Consider combination therapy with fibrates or nicotinic acid plus a statin.

Low-dose ASA for patients at intermediate and high risk.

Source: Circulation 2004;109:551–556.

DEPRESSION: MANAGEMENT

OVERVIEW OF TREATMENT FOR DEPRESSION
Source: AHRQ

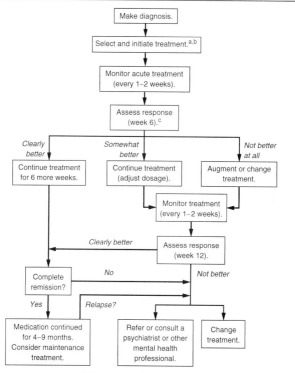

[a]ACP guidelines recommend either tricyclic antidepressants or newer antidepressants, such as selective serotonin reuptake inhibitors, as equally efficacious. (Ann Intern Med 2000;132:738)

[b]Treating depression effectively leads to improved comorbidity-associated pain control and functional status (e.g., arthritis, diabetes). (JAMA 2003;290:2428; Ann Intern Med 2004;140:1015)

[c]Times of assessment (weeks 6 and 12) rest on very modest data. It may be necessary to revise the treatment plan earlier for patients who fail to respond at all.

Source: Reproduced, with permission, from the AHRQ: Depression in Primary Care. Vol. 2: Treatment of Major Depression. United States Department of Health and Human Services, 1993.

DIABETES MELLITUS: MANAGEMENT

MANAGEMENT OF HYPERGLYCEMIA[a]
Source: ADA

```
┌──────────────┐
│ All diabetics │
└──────────────┘
        │
        ▼
┌─────────────────────────────────────┐
│ • Appropriate frequency of self-monitored │
│   blood glucose (SMBG) determinations │
│ • Medical nutrition therapy           │
│ • Regular physical activity program    │
│ • Recognition, prevention, and treatment │
│   of hypoglycemia symptoms            │
│ • Periodic assessment of treatment goals │
└─────────────────────────────────────┘
```

```
        Type 1                    Type 2
          │                         │
          ▼                         ▼
┌─────────────────────┐   ┌──────────────────────────┐
│ Physiologically based │   │ Step Care: oral agent →   │
│ insulin replacement   │   │ add nocturnal insulin →   │
│                       │   │ ↑ insulin as needed to achieve │
│                       │   │ treatment goals           │
└─────────────────────┘   └──────────────────────────┘
```

```
        ┌──────────────────┐
        │ Treatment Goals[b] │
        └──────────────────┘
                │
                ▼
┌─────────────────────────────────────────────────┐
│ • SMBG:  90–130 mg/dL before meals                │
│          < 180 mg/dL 1.5–2.0 hours postprandially │
│ • HbA$_{1c}$: < 7.0%[c]                            │
└─────────────────────────────────────────────────┘
```

[a]Diabetes defined as fasting blood glucose ≥126 mg/dL, or random glucose >200 mg/dL in person with symptoms of diabetes; these criteria should be confirmed by repeat testing on a different day.

[b]These are generalized goals. They do not apply to pregnant adults. One should modify individual treatment goals to take into account risk for hypoglycemia, very young or old age, end-stage renal disease, advanced cardiovascular or cerebrovascular disease, or other diseases that decrease life expectancy.

[c]More stringent goals (i.e., <6%) can be considered in some patients.

Source: ADA Diabetes Care 2004;27(Suppl 1).

PREVENTION & TREATMENT OF DIABETIC COMPLICATIONS/COMORBIDITIES
Source: ADA

PREVENTION & TREATMENT OF DIABETIC COMPLICATIONS/COMORBIDITIES

Complication or Comorbidity	Goal	Monitoring/Treatment	Action if Goal Not Met
Hyperglycemia[a]	$HbA_{1c} < 7.0\%$[b] Preprandial plasma glucose 90–130 mg/dL. Peak postprandial plasma glucose < 180 mg/dL	HbA_{1c} = every 6 months if meeting treatment goals; every 3 months in those not meeting goals.	See management, previous page.
Retinopathy	Prevent vision loss	Optimize glycemic and blood pressure control. Annual retinal exam.[c]	Laser treatment
Neuropathy	Prevent foot complications	Annual foot exam[d] and visual inspection at every visit.	Refer high-risk patients to a foot care specialist.
Nephropathy	Prevent renal failure	Optimize glucose and blood pressure control. Annual urinary protein determination (see next page). Spot albumin: creatinine testing preferred. Continued surveillance even if treated with ACE or ARB.	See below[e] for treatment; consider nephrology referral.
Hypertension	Adult: BP < 130/80[f] mm Hg	Every routine diabetes visit.[g]	See JNC VII, page 117. If ACEs or adrenergic receptor binders are used, monitor renal function and potassium levels.

PREVENTION & TREATMENT OF DIABETIC COMPLICATIONS/COMORBIDITIES
Source: ADA

PREVENTION & TREATMENT OF DIABETIC COMPLICATIONS/COMORBIDITIES (CONTINUED)

Complication or Comorbidity	Goal	Monitoring/Treatment	Action if Goal Not Met
Hyperlipidemia	LDL < 100 mg/dL TG < 150 mg/dL HDL > 40 mg/dL	Annual determination, and more frequently to achieve goals. If low-risk (LDL < 100, HDL > 60, TG < 150), then assess every 2 years. Routine monitoring of liver and muscle enzymes in asymptomatic patients is not recommended unless patient has baseline enzyme abnormalities or is taking drugs that interact with statins. (ACP; Ann Intern Med 2004;140:644).	Weight loss; increase in physical activity; nutrition therapy; follow NCEP recommendations for pharmacologic treatment, Appendix VII
Macrovascular disease	Prevent limb ischemia, stroke, and MI	1) Use aspirin therapy (75–162 mg/day) as primary prevention for all patients ≥ 40 years or those with ≥ 1 cardiovascular risk factor if age 21–39 years. 2) Smoking cessation. 3) Manage hyperlipidemia and hypertension as above. 4) Assess for peripheral arterial disease with pedal pulses ± ankle brachial pressure index via doppler.	

[a]Less intensive glycemic goals if severe or frequent hypoglycemia.
[b]Postprandial glucose may be targeted if HbA$_{1c}$ goals are not met despite meeting preprandial goals.
[c]Dilated eye exam or 7-field 30-degree fundus photography by ophthalmologist or optometrist. In setting of normal eye exam, less frequent screening can be considered by eye specialist.
[d]Includes evaluation of protective sensation (monofilament test and tuning fork), vascular status, and inspection for foot deformities or ulcers.
[e]Microalbuminuria treatment: if type 1, use ACE inhibitor; if type 2 and hypertensive, use ACE or ARB. Clinical albuminuria treatment: (1) Achieve BP < 130/80 mm Hg; (2) use ACE inhibitor or ARB; (3) tight glycemic control; and (4) decrease protein to 10% of dietary intake, especially in patients progressing despite optimal glucose and BP control. Refer to nephrologist if: estimated glomerular filtration rate < 30 mg/minute, creatinine > 2.0 mg/dL, or when management of hypertension or hyperkalemia is difficult.
[f]ALLHAT trial showed no difference in cardiovascular and renal outcomes in diabetes treated with diuretics or ACE (or ARB). (JAMA 2002;288:2981) Diuretics should be first line in black patients. (Ann Intern Med 2003;138:587)
[g]ACP recommends tight BP control (SBP < 135, DBP < 80).
Source: Adapted from American Diabetes Association Position Statement "Standards of Medical Care for Patients With Diabetes Mellitus." Last updated January 2004. (http://www.diabetes.org/for-health-professionals-and-scientists/cpr.jsp)

PREVENTION & TREATMENT OF DIABETIC COMPLICATIONS/COMORBIDITIES
Source: **ADA**

PREVENTION & TREATMENT OF DIABETIC COMPLICATIONS/COMORBIDITIES (CONTINUED)

Category	Albuminuria Thresholds		
	24-hour collection (mg/24 hour)	Timed collection (µg/minute)	Spot collection (albumin: creatinine ratio) (µg/mg)[a]
Normal	< 30	< 20	< 30
Microalbuminuria	30–299	20–200	30–299
Clinical (macro) albuminuria	≥ 300	> 200	≥ 300

Because of variability in urinary albumin excretion, 2 of 3 specimens collected within a 3- to 6-month period should be abnormal before considering a patient to have crossed one of these diagnostic thresholds. Exercise within 24 hours, infection, fever, congestive heart failure, marked hyperglycemia, and marked hypertension may elevate urinary albumin excretion over baseline values.
[a]Strongly encouraged as preferred test.
Source: ADA

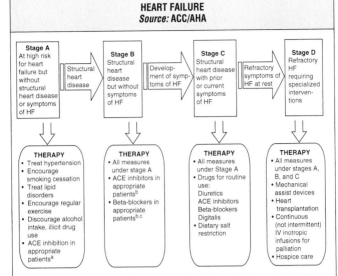

HEART FAILURE
Source: ACC/AHA

Stage A: Patients with hypertension, coronary artery disease, diabetes mellitus *or* those using cardiotoxins or having a FHx CM

Stage B: Patients with previous MI, LV systolic dysfunction, or asymptomatic valvular disease

Stage C: Patients with known structural heart disease; shortness of breath and fatigue, reduced exercise tolerance

Stage D: Patients who have marked symptoms at rest despite maximal medical therapy (eg, those who are recurrently hospitalized or cannot be safely discharged from hospital without specialized interventions)

Footnotes:

[a]History of atherosclerotic vascular disease, diabetes mellitus, or hypertension and associated cardiovascular risk factors.

[b]Recent or remote MI, regardless of ejection fraction; or reduced ejection fraction.

[c]Compared with placebo, beta-blocker use is associated with a consistent 30% reduction in mortality and 40% reduction in hospitalizations in patients with class II and III heart failure. (JAMA 2002;287:883)

Comments: 1) Implementing a CHF disease management program for patients with ejection fractions < 20% was associated with decreased hospitalizations. (Arch Intern Med 2001;161:2223) 2) Exercise training in patients with HF seems to be safe and beneficial overall in improving exercise capacity, quality of life, muscle structure, and physiologic responses to exercise. (Circulation 2003;107:1210–1225)

FHx CM = family history of cardiomyopathy; HF = heart failure; LV = left ventricle

Source: Adapted and reproduced with permission from the American College of Cardiology and American Heart Association, Inc. J Am Coll Cardiol 2001;38:2101.

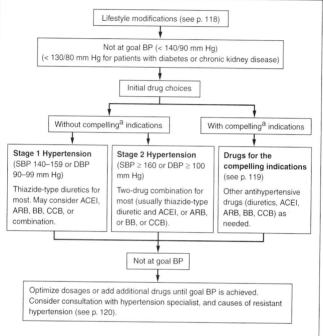

HYPERTENSION: INITIATING TREATMENT
Source: **The 7th Report of the Joint National Committee on Prevention, Detection, Evaluation and Treatment of High Blood Pressure**

Lifestyle modifications (see p. 118)

Not at goal BP (< 140/90 mm Hg)
(< 130/80 mm Hg for patients with diabetes or chronic kidney disease)

Initial drug choices

Without compelling[a] indications

With compelling[a] indications

Stage 1 Hypertension
(SBP 140–159 or DBP 90–99 mm Hg)

Thiazide-type diuretics for most. May consider ACEI, ARB, BB, CCB, or combination.

Stage 2 Hypertension
(SBP ≥ 160 or DBP ≥ 100 mm Hg)

Two-drug combination for most (usually thiazide-type diuretic and ACEI, or ARB, or BB, or CCB).

Drugs for the compelling indications
(see p. 119)

Other antihypertensive drugs (diuretics, ACEI, ARB, BB, CCB) as needed.

Not at goal BP

Optimize dosages or add additional drugs until goal BP is achieved. Consider consultation with hypertension specialist, and causes of resistant hypertension (see p. 120).

Drug abbreviations: ACEI, ACE inhibitor; ARB, angiotensin receptor blocker; BB, beta-blocker; CCB, calcium channel blocker.

[a]Compelling indications: CHF, high coronary disease risk, diabetes, chronic kidney disease, recurrent stroke prevention.

Source: JNC VII, 2003. (Hypertension 2003;42:1206–1252)

LIFESTYLE MODIFICATIONS FOR PRIMARY PREVENTION OF HYPERTENSION[a,b]

Modification	Recommendation	Approximate SBP Reduction (Range)
Weight reduction	Maintain normal body weight (BMI 18.5–24.9 kg/m^2).	5–20 mm Hg per 10 kg weight loss
Adopt DASH eating plan	Consume diet rich in fruits, vegetables, and low fat dairy products with a reduced content of saturated and total fat.	8–14 mm Hg
Dietary sodium reduction	Reduce dietary sodium intake to no more than 100 mmol/day (2.4 g sodium or 6 g sodium chloride).	2–8 mm Hg
Physical activity	Engage in regular aerobic physical activity such as brisk walking (at least 30 min/day, most days of the week).	4–9 mm Hg
Moderation of alcohol consumption	Limit consumption to no more than 2 drinks (1 oz or 30 mL ethanol; eg, 24 oz beer, 10 oz wine, or 3 oz 80-proof whiskey) per day in most men and to no more than 1 drink per day in women and lighter-weight persons.	2–4 mm Hg

[a]For overall cardiovascular risk reduction, stop smoking.
[b]The effects of implementing these modifications are dose and time dependent and could be greater for some individuals.
DASH = Dietary Approaches to Stop Hypertension

RECOMMENDED MEDICATIONS FOR COMPELLING INDICATIONS

Compelling Indication[b]	Recommended Medications[a]					
	Diuretic	BB	ACEI	ARB	CCB	AldoANT
Heart failure	X	X	X	X		X
Post-MI		X	X			X
High coronary disease risk	X	X	X		X	
Diabetes	X	X	X	X	X	
Chronic kidney disease			X	X		
Recurrent stroke prevention	X		X			

[a]Drug abbreviations: ACEI, ACE inhibitor; ARB, angiotensin receptor blocker; AldoANT, aldosterone antagonist; BB, beta-blocker; CCB, calcium channel blocker.
[b]Compelling indications for antihypertensive drugs are based on benefits from outcome studies or existing clinical guidelines; the compelling indication is managed in parallel with the BP.

CAUSES OF RESISTANT HYPERTENSION

Improper BP Measurement
Volume Overload and Pseudotolerance
Excess sodium intake
Volume retention from kidney disease
Inadequate diuretic therapy
Drug-Induced or Other Causes
Nonadherence
Inadequate doses
Inappropriate combinations
Nonsteroidal anti-inflammatory drugs; cyclooxygenase 2 inhibitors
Cocaine, amphetamines, other illicit drugs
Sympathomimetics (decongestants, anoretics)
Oral contraceptives
Adrenal steroids
Cyclosporine and tacrolimus
Erythropoietin
Licorice (including some chewing tobacco)
Select over-the-counter dietary supplements and medicines (eg, ephedra, mahuang, bitter orange)
Associated Conditions
Obesity
Excess alcohol intake
Identifiable Causes
Sleep apnea
Chronic kidney disease
Primary aldosteronism
Renovascular disease
Steroid excess (Cushing syndrome; chronic steroid therapy)
Pheochromocytoma
Coarctation of aorta
Thyroid or parathyroid disease
Obstructive uropathy

ADULT ACUTE LOW BACK PAIN: ALGORITHM 1. INITIAL EVALUATION
Sources: Agency for Healthcare Research and Quality; American Academy of
Family Practitioners; American College of Radiology; American Academy of
Orthopedic Surgeons

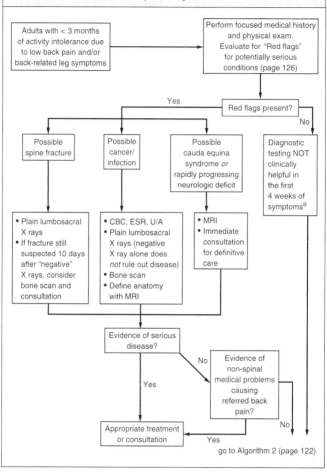

go to Algorithm 2 (page 122)

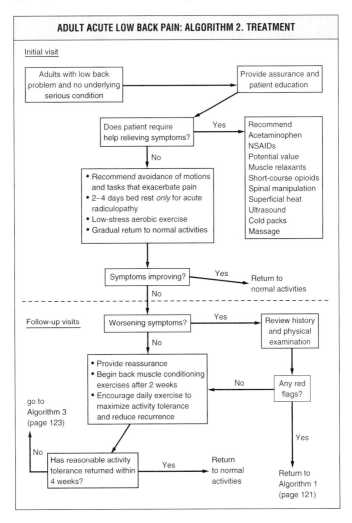

ADULT ACUTE LOW BACK PAIN: ALGORITHM 2. TREATMENT

Initial visit

Adults with low back problem and no underlying serious condition → Provide assurance and patient education

Does patient require help relieving symptoms? — Yes → Recommend Acetaminophen NSAIDs Potential value Muscle relaxants Short-course opioids Spinal manipulation Superficial heat Ultrasound Cold packs Massage

No

- Recommend avoidance of motions and tasks that exacerbate pain
- 2–4 days bed rest *only* for acute radiculopathy
- Low-stress aerobic exercise
- Gradual return to normal activities

Symptoms improving? — Yes → Return to normal activities

No

Follow-up visits — Worsening symptoms? — Yes → Review history and physical examination

No

- Provide reassurance
- Begin back muscle conditioning exercises after 2 weeks
- Encourage daily exercise to maximize activity tolerance and reduce recurrence

Any red flags? — No →

Yes

go to Algorithm 3 (page 123)

No

Has reasonable activity tolerance returned within 4 weeks? — Yes → Return to normal activities

Return to Algorithm 1 (page 121)

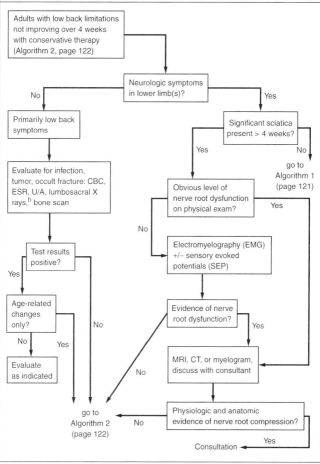

**ADULT ACUTE LOW BACK PAIN: ALGORITHM 3.
EVALUATION OF SLOW-TO-RECOVER PATIENT (SYMPTOMS > 4 WEEKS)**

Adults with low back limitations not improving over 4 weeks with conservative therapy (Algorithm 2, page 122)

Neurologic symptoms in lower limb(s)?

No — Primarily low back symptoms

Evaluate for infection, tumor, occult fracture: CBC, ESR, U/A, lumbosacral X rays,[b] bone scan

Test results positive?

Yes — Age-related changes only?

No — Evaluate as indicated

Yes — go to Algorithm 2 (page 122)

No — go to Algorithm 2 (page 122)

Yes — Significant sciatica present > 4 weeks?

No — go to Algorithm 1 (page 121)

Yes — Obvious level of nerve root dysfunction on physical exam?

No — Electromyelography (EMG) +/− sensory evoked potentials (SEP)

Evidence of nerve root dysfunction?

No — go to Algorithm 2 (page 122)

Yes — MRI, CT, or myelogram, discuss with consultant

Yes — MRI, CT, or myelogram, discuss with consultant

Physiologic and anatomic evidence of nerve root compression?

No — go to Algorithm 2 (page 122)

Yes — Consultation

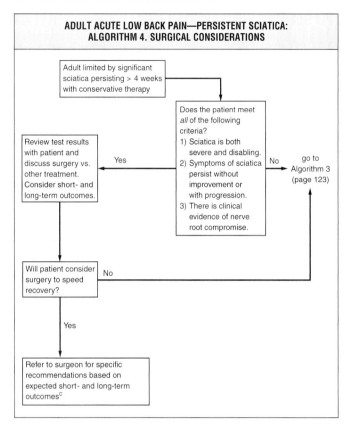

ADULT ACUTE LOW BACK PAIN—PERSISTENT SCIATICA: ALGORITHM 4. SURGICAL CONSIDERATIONS

Adult limited by significant sciatica persisting > 4 weeks with conservative therapy

Does the patient meet *all* of the following criteria?
1) Sciatica is both severe and disabling.
2) Symptoms of sciatica persist without improvement or with progression.
3) There is clinical evidence of nerve root compromise.

No → go to Algorithm 3 (page 123)

Yes → Review test results with patient and discuss surgery vs. other treatment. Consider short- and long-term outcomes.

Will patient consider surgery to speed recovery?

No →

Yes ↓

Refer to surgeon for specific recommendations based on expected short- and long-term outcomes[c]

[a]**Footnote to Algorithm 1:**

It has generally been believed that 80%–90% of acute low back pain episodes recover spontaneously within 4 weeks. However, more recent studies indicate that there may be a significant percentage of individuals who continue to have pain or functional limitation at 1 year. Recurrences are common, affecting 40% of patients within 6 months. The emerging picture is that of a chronic problem with intermittent exacerbations, rather than an acute disease that can be cured.

Sources:

J Gen Intern Med 2001;16:120–131, N Engl J Med 2001;244:363–370, Spine 1996;21:2900–2907, BMJ 1998;316:1356–1359, BMJ 1999;318:1662–1667.

[b]**Footnote to Algorithm 3:**

In an RCT, MRIs and radiographs resulted in nearly identical outcomes for primary care patients with low back pain. Substituting MRI for radiographs in the primary care setting may offer little additional benefit to patients and may increase the cost of care. (JAMA 2003;289:2810–2818)

[c]**Footnote to Algorithm 4:**

Herniated disk: Surgery for herniated disks is invasive and comprises all types of surgical and injection techniques to remove or reduce the size of herniated intervertebral disks that compress nerve roots. Included are standard discectomy, microscopic discectomy, percutaneous discectomy, and chemonucleolysis. The therapeutic objective is to relieve pressure on nerve roots and reduce pain and possibly weakness and/or numbness in the lower extremities. Lumbar discectomy may relieve symptoms faster than continued nonsurgical therapy in patients who have severe and disabling leg symptoms and who have not improved after 4–8 weeks of adequate nonsurgical treatment. However, in nonemergent patients, there appears to be little difference in long-term outcomes at 4 and 10 years between discectomy and conservative care.

Spinal stenosis: Elderly patients with spinal stenosis who can adequately function in the activities of daily life can be managed with conservative treatments. Surgery for spinal stenosis should not usually be considered in the first 3 months of symptoms. Decisions on treatment should take into account the patient's lifestyle, preference, other medical problems, and risk of surgery. In one study of patients with severe lumbar spinal stenosis, surgical treatment was associated with greater improvement in patient-reported outcomes than nonsurgical treatment at 4 years (70% vs. 52% reported that their predominant symptom was better). The relative benefit of surgery declined over time but remained superior to nonsurgical treatment. (Spine 2000;25:556–562)

USPSTF: Insufficient evidence to recommend for or against routine use of interventions to prevent low back pain in adults in primary care settings (2004).

Sources:

Bigos S et al. Acute low back problems in adults. Rockville, MD: U.S. Department of Health and Human Services, Public Health Service, Agency for Health Care Policy and Research, 1994. AHCPR Publication no. 95-0642. Patel AT, Oble AA. Diagnosis and Management of Acute Low Back Pain. Am Fam Physician 2000;61:1779–86. American College of Radiology. ACR Appropriateness Criteria (http://www.acr.org, website accessed 7/23/04). American Academy of Orthopedic Surgeons Clinical Guideline on Low Back Pain (http://www.aaos.org, website accessed 7/23/04).

RED FLAGS FOR POTENTIALLY SERIOUS CONDITIONS

	Fracture	Cancer or Infection	Cauda Equina Syndrome
History Features			
Major trauma, ie, motor vehicle accident or fall from height	X		
Minor trauma or strenuous lifting (older or osteoporotic patient)	X		
Age > 50 or < 20		X	
History of cancer		X	
Constitutional symptoms (ie, fever, weight loss)		X	
Risk factors for spinal infection (ie, recent bacterial infection, IV drug use, immune suppression)		X	
Pain that worsens when supine		X	
Severe nighttime pain		X	
Saddle anesthesia			X
Recent onset of bladder dysfunction (ie, urinary retention, increased frequency, overflow incontinence)			X
Severe or progressive lower extremity neurologic deficit			X
Physical Examination Features			
Anal sphincter laxity			X
Perianal/perineal sensory loss			X
Major motor weakness: knee extension, foot drop			X

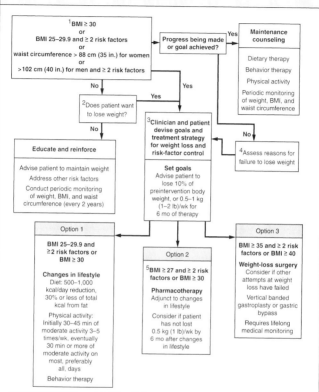

OBESITY MANAGEMENT: ADULTS
Source: NHLBI

[¹]BMI ≥ 30
or
BMI 25–29.9 and ≥ 2 risk factors
or
waist circumference > 88 cm (35 in.) for women
or
>102 cm (40 in.) for men and ≥ 2 risk factors

Progress being made or goal achieved? — Yes →

Maintenance counseling
Dietary therapy
Behavior therapy
Physical activity
Periodic monitoring of weight, BMI, and waist circumference

No ↓

[²]Does patient want to lose weight? — Yes →

[³]Clinician and patient devise goals and treatment strategy for weight loss and risk-factor control

No ↓

Educate and reinforce
Advise patient to maintain weight
Address other risk factors
Conduct periodic monitoring of weight, BMI, and waist circumference (every 2 years)

No → [⁴]Assess reasons for failure to lose weight

Set goals
Advise patient to lose 10% of preintervention body weight, or 0.5–1 kg (1–2 lb)/wk for 6 mo of therapy

Option 1

BMI 25–29.9 and ≥ 2 risk factors or BMI ≥ 30

Changes in lifestyle
Diet: 500–1,000 kcal/day reduction, 30% or less of total kcal from fat
Physical activity: Initially 30–45 min of moderate activity 3–5 times/wk, eventually 30 min or more of moderate activity on most, preferably all, days
Behavior therapy

Option 2

[⁵]BMI ≥ 27 and ≥ 2 risk factors or BMI ≥ 30

Pharmacotherapy
Adjunct to changes in lifestyle
Consider if patient has not lost 0.5 kg (1 lb)/wk by 6 mo after changes in lifestyle

Option 3

BMI ≥ 35 and ≥ 2 risk factors or BMI ≥ 40

Weight-loss surgery
Consider if other attempts at weight loss have failed
Vertical banded gastroplasty or gastric bypass
Requires lifelong medical monitoring

Notes for Obesity Management Guideline: Adults

1. Risk factors: cigarette smoking; hypertension or current use of antihypertensive agents; LDL cholesterol ≥ 160 mg/dL or LDL cholesterol 130–159 mg/dL+ ≥ 2 other risk factors; HDL cholesterol < 35 mg/dL; fasting plasma glucose 110–125 mg/dL; family history of premature CHD (MI or sudden death in 1st degree ♂ relative ≤ 55 years old or 1st degree ♀ relative ≤ 65 years old; age ≥ 45 for ♂ or ≥ 55 years for ♀.
2. The decision to lose weight must be made in the context of other risk factors (eg, quitting smoking is more important than losing weight).
3. The decision to lose weight must be made jointly between the clinician and the patient.
4. Investigate: patient's level of motivation; energy intake (dietary recall); energy expenditure (physical activity diary); attendance at psychological/behavioral counseling sessions; recent negative life events; family and societal pressures; evidence of detrimental psychiatric problems (eg, depression, binge eating disorder).
5. Pharmacotherapy should be considered as an adjunct only for patients who are at substantial medical risk because of their obesity and in whom nonpharmacologic treatments have not resulted in sufficient weight loss to improve health. The safety and efficacy of weight-loss medications beyond 2 years of use have not been established. Two medications available for long-term use: sibutramine (5–15 mg/day) and/or orlistat (120 mg 3 times/day with or within 1 hour after fat-containing meals, plus a daily multivitamin).

Source: Adapted from the National Institutes of Health. NEJM 2002;346[8]:591–599; http://www.nhlbi. nih.gov/guidelines/obesity/ob_home.htm

OBESITY MANAGEMENT: CHILDREN
Source: Expert Committee, Department of Health and Human Services

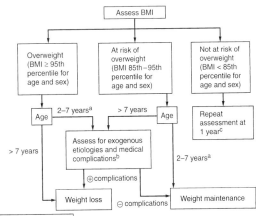

Approach to therapy:

1. Begin interventions early—risk of persistent obesity increases with age of child.
2. Family must be ready to change—defer treatment until family ready or refer to therapist.
3. Educate families about medical complications of obesity.
4. Involve family and *all* caregivers in treatment program.
5. Institute permanent changes—methodic, gradual, long-term changes will be more successful than multiple, frequent changes.
6. Family should learn to monitor eating and activity.
7. Recommend 2–3 specific changes in diet or activity at a time—additional recommendations only after success.
8. Emphasize successful behavior changes rather than weight loss; empathize with struggles experienced.
9. Utilize a team approach; consider group meetings.
10. Provide guidance in parenting skills—avoid using food as a reward; offer only healthy options; be a role model.
11. Increase activity level: limit television, incorporate activity into usual daily activities, aim for ≥ 30 minutes of activity on most days.
12. Reduce calorie intake: identify and eliminate high-calorie foods.
13. Stop tobacco use (adolescents).

Footnotes:

[a]Children younger than 2 years should be referred to a pediatric obesity center.
[b]Evaluate for: 1. Exogenous causes: genetic syndromes, hypothyroidism, Cushing's syndrome, eating disorders, depression; 2. Complications: hypertension, dyslipidemias, noninsulin-dependent diabetes mellitus, slipped capital femoral epiphysis, pseudotumor cerebri, sleep apnea or obesity hypoventilation syndrome, gallbladder disease, polycystic ovary disease.
[c]Use change in BMI to identify rate of excessive weight gain relative to linear growth.

Source: Pediatrics 1998;102(3) (http://pediatrics.aapublications.org/cgi/content/full/102/3/e29); Pediatrics 2003;112:424–430.

OSTEOPOROSIS: MANAGEMENT[c]
Source: American Academy of Clinical Endocrinologists

Known osteoporotic fracture or osteoporosis by DXA[a]

Treatment for all:
- Calcium supplementation 1,000–1,500 mg/day
- Vitamin D 400–800 IU/day
- Weight-bearing exercise 30 min/day, 3 d/wk
- Strongly discourage tobacco
- Avoid glucocorticoids
- Hip protectors if high fall risk

+

Pharmacologic Management[b]

Agents approved for treatment of osteoporosis:
- Bisphosphonates (alendronate, risedronate)
  - ↑ BMD of spine, hip and ↓ vertebral and nonvertebral fracture risk
- Calcitonin
  - ↓ vertebral but *not* nonvertebral fracture risk
  - Modest ↑ spinal BMD
  - Analgesic effect in acute osteoporotic fracture
- Estrogen
  - Must individualize risk/benefit assessment
  - ↓ vertebral and hip fracture risk
- Selective estrogen receptor modulators (SERMs—Raloxifene)
  - Modest ↑ BMD spine and hip
  - ↓ vertebral fracture risk
  - No documented ↓ in nonvertebral fracture risk
- Parathyroid Hormone (Teriparatide)
  - Subcutaneous injection
  - ↓ risk of vertebral and nonvertebral fractures
- Combination Therapy (bisphosphate + non-bisphosphate)
  - Can provide additional small ↑ BMD vs. monotherapy
  - Impact on fracture risk unknown

[a]Indications for treatment
- ♀ with T scores below ≤–2.5 in the absence of risk factors
- ♀ with T scores –1.5 to –2.5 if other risk factors present (see page 54)
- Prior vertebral or hip fracture

[b]Selection of pharmacologic agents for treating osteoporosis should be based on individual risk/benefit and preferences. Bisphosphanates are indicated for male osteoporosis and for glucocorticoid-induced osteoporosis.

[c]Follow-up: perform follow-up BMD yearly for 2 years. If bone mass stabilizes after 2 years, remeasure every 2 years. Otherwise, continue annual BMD until bone mass is stable. Medicare covers BMD every 2 years. Biochemical markers of BME turnover can be used to monitor response to treatment.

Source: Adapted from AACE 2003 Medical Guidelines for Clinical Practice for the Prevention and Management of Postmenopausal Osteoporosis, and NOF guidelines for treatment (www.nof.org, website accessed 10/18/03).

PALLIATIVE AND END-OF-LIFE CARE: HOSPICE ELIGIBILITY

ELIGIBILITY CRITERIA FOR THE MEDICARE HOSPICE BENEFIT

Patient is eligible for Medicare Part A.

Usually anyone who is 65 years of age or older, or who is on hemodialysis or receives Medicare disability payments, is eligible.

Patient is terminally ill.

Two physicians must sign a statement certifying that the patient's medical prognosis is 6 months or less, if the disease runs its normal course. One of the physicians must be the hospice medical director or the hospice team physician; the other must be the patient's attending physician. When the hospice medical director serves as the patient's attending physician, only the signature of the medical director is required.

Patient chooses hospice care (informed consent).

The patient chooses hospice care and signs a Medicare hospice benefit election form, understanding that the goals of care are palliative rather than curative.

Care is provided by a Medicare-certified hospice program.

All care for the terminal illness is provided by a Medicare-certified hospice program.

Reprinted with permission from the American Academy of Hospice and Palliative Medicine. *Pocket Guide to Hospice/Palliative Medicine.*

PALLIATIVE AND END-OF-LIFE CARE: HOSPICE ELIGIBILITY

COMPARISON OF THE MEDICARE HOSPICE AND MEDICARE HOME CARE BENEFITS

	Medicare Hospice	**Medicare Home Health Care**
Patient must be homebound.	No	Yes
Service Provided		
100% coverage of medications to control pain and other symptoms related to the terminal illness (hospice programs can charge a 5% copayment).	Yes	No
100% coverage of durable medical equipment and medical supplies without a deductible or copayment.	Yes	No
Homemakers/home health aides.	Yes	Yes
Inpatient respite care (hospice programs can charge a 5% copayment).	Yes	No
Inpatient care with no deductible.	Yes	No
Continuous registered nurse care in the home during periods of medical crisis.	Yes	No
Counseling in the home for patient/family.	Yes	Limited
Bereavement support.	Yes	No
Trained volunteers.	Yes	No
Professional management and supervision of care in all settings, including inpatient.	Yes	No
Ongoing pastoral counseling and spiritual support for patients and family.	Yes	No
Payment of consulting physician fees at 100% of Medicare allowance.	Yes	No
Physician, nurse, social worker, and counselor on-call availability 24 hours a day, 7 days a week.	Yes	No

Reprinted with permission from the American Academy of Hospice and Palliative Medicine. *Pocket Guide to Hospice/Palliative Medicine.*

PALLIATIVE AND END-OF-LIFE CARE: HOSPICE ELIGIBILITY

SUMMARY OF THE NATIONAL HOSPICE ORGANIZATION'S GUIDELINES FOR DETERMINING PROGNOSIS OF 6 MONTHS OR LESS[a]

Disease	Primary Factors	Secondary Factors
Heart disease	Symptoms of recurrent heart failure or angina at rest, discomfort with any activity (NYHA Class IV) Patient already optimally treated with diuretics and vasodilators (eg, angiotensin-converting enzyme inhibitors)	Ejection fraction $\leq 20\%$ Symptomatic arrhythmias History of cardiac arrest and CPR Unexplained syncope Embolic cerebrovascular accident of cardiac origin HIV disease
Pulmonary disease	Disabling dyspnea at rest Progressive pulmonary disease (eg, increasing emergency room visits or hospitalizations for pulmonary infections and/or respiratory failure) Hypoxemia at rest on supplemental O_2 $pO_2 \leq 55$ mm Hg on supplemental O_2 O_2 sat $\leq 88\%$ on supplemental O_2 OR Hypercapnia $pCO_2 \geq 50$ mm Hg	FEV1 after bronchodilator $< 30\%$ of predicted for normal patients Decreased FEV1 on serial testing > 40 mL per year Unintentional weight loss $> 10\%$ of body weight in 6 months Resting tachycardia > 100 beats/minute in patient with severe chronic obstructive pulmonary disease Documented cor pulmonale or right heart failure due to advanced pulmonary disease
Dementia	Severity of dementia $\geq$ FAST Stage 7-C Unable to walk, dress, or bathe without assistance Urinary and fecal incontinence Unable to speak more than six different intelligible words per day Severe comorbid condition within past 6 months Aspiration pneumonia Pyelonephritis Septicemia Multiple, progressive stage 3–4 decubiti Fever after antibiotics Unable to maintain fluid/caloric intake to sustain life If feeding tube in place, weight loss $> 10\%$ in 6 months or serum albumin < 2.5 g/dL	

PALLIATIVE AND END-OF-LIFE CARE: HOSPICE ELIGIBILITY

SUMMARY OF THE NATIONAL HOSPICE ORGANIZATION'S GUIDELINES FOR DETERMINING PROGNOSIS OF 6 MONTHS OR LESS[a] (CONTINUED)

Disease	Primary Factors	Secondary Factors

HIV disease (Developed prior to highly active antiretroviral therapies.)	CD4+ < 25 cells/mL
	OR
	Viral load ≥ 100,000 copies/mL
	Karnofsky ≤ 50%
	One of the following:
	    Central nervous system lymphoma
	    Progressive multifocal leukoencephalopathy
	    Advanced dementia
	    Cryptosporidiosis
	    Wasting > 33% of body weight
	    Toxoplasmosis
	    Visceral Kaposi's sarcoma, no Rx
	    Mycobacterium avium complex, no Rx
	    Renal failure, no dialysis
		Foregoing antiretroviral and prophylactic drug Rx
		Chronic, persistent diarrhea for 1 year
		Albumin < 2.5 g/dL
		Age > 50 years
		CHF, NYHA Class IV
		Active substance abuse
		Note: A Karnofsky performance score ≤ 50% indicates the patient requires considerable assistance and frequent medical care.

Liver disease	End-stage cirrhosis; not a candidate for liver transplant
	Prothrombin time > 5 seconds over control or INR > 1.5 AND serum albumin < 2.5 g/dL
	At least one of the following:
	    Ascites despite diuretics and low-sodium diet
	    Spontaneous bacterial peritonitis
	    Hepatorenal syndrome
	    Hepatic encephalopathy despite treatment
	    Recurrent variceal bleed
		Progressive malnutrition
		Muscle wasting
		Continued alcoholism
		Primary liver cancer
		Positive HbsAg

Renal disease	Chronic renal failure; coming off or not a candidate for dialysis
	Creatinine clearance < 10 cc/minute (for diabetics < 15 cc/minute) AND serum creatinine > 8.0 mg/dL (for diabetics, > 6.0 mg/dL)
	Signs and symptoms associated with renal failure:
	    Uremia: nausea, pruritus, confusion, or restlessness
	    Oliguria: output < 400 cc/24 hours
	    Intractable hyperkalemia: serum K > 7.0
	    Uremic pericarditis
	    Hepatorenal syndrome
	    Intractable fluid overload
		Mechanical ventilation
		Malignancy—other organ system
		Chronic lung disease
		Advanced cardiac or liver disease
		Sepsis
		Cachexia or albumin ≤ 3.5 g/dL
		Age > 75 years
		Platelets < 25,000
		Gastrointestinal bleed
		Disseminated intravascular coagulation

PALLIATIVE AND END-OF-LIFE CARE: HOSPICE ELIGIBILITY

SUMMARY OF THE NATIONAL HOSPICE ORGANIZATION'S GUIDELINES FOR DETERMINING PROGNOSIS OF 6 MONTHS OR LESS[a] (CONTINUED)

Disease	Primary Factors	Secondary Factors

Stroke and coma	*Acute phase after cerebrovascular accident*
	Coma or persistent vegetative state > 3 days
	Any one of the following on day 3 of coma:
	    Abnormal brain stem response
	    Absent verbal response
	    Absent withdrawal to pain
	    Serum creatine > 1.5 mg/dL
	Inability to maintain fluid/caloric intake to sustain life
	Chronic phase of cerebrovascular accident
	Any one of the following:
	    Age > 70 years
	    Poststroke dementia: FAST score > 7 (unable to toilet, dress, or bathe without assistance; unable to speak more than 6 different intelligible words per day; and occasional urinary or fecal incontinence)
	    Karnofsky ≤ 50%
	    Poor nutritional status
		Aspiration pneumonia
		Upper urinary tract infection (eg, pyelonephritis)
		Sepsis
		Progressive, refractory stage 3–4 decubiti
		Fever after antibiotics
		Note: A Karnofsky score ≤ 50% indicates the patient requires considerable assistance and frequent medical care.

[a]A life-limiting condition with evidence of either disease progression and/or impaired nutritional status indicated by involuntary weight loss ≥ 10% of body weight in past 6 months. Serum albumin ≤ 2.5 is a helpful but not necessary factor. The goal of treatment is relief of symptoms, not cure.
Source: Summarized with permission from the National Hospice and Palliative Care Organization. All rights reserved.

PALLIATIVE AND END-OF-LIFE CARE: PAIN MANAGEMENT

PRINCIPLES OF ANALGESIC USE

By the mouth	The oral route is the preferred route for analgesics, including morphine.
By the clock	Persistent pain requires around-the-clock treatment to prevent further pain. PRN dosing is irrational and inhumane; it requires patients to experience pain before becoming eligible for relief.
By the WHO ladder	If a maximum dose of medication fails to adequately relieve pain, move up the ladder, not laterally to a different drug in the same efficiency group. Severe pain requires immediate use of an opioid recommended for controlling severe pain, without progressing sequentially through Steps 1 and 2.
Individualize treatment	The right dose of an analgesic is the dose that relieves pain with acceptable side effects for a specific patient.
Monitor	Monitoring is required to ensure the benefits of treatment are maximized while adverse effects are minimized.
Use adjuvant drugs	For example, an NSAID is almost always needed to help control bone pain. Nonopioid analgesics, such as NSAIDs or acetaminophen, can be used at any step of the ladder. Adjuvant medications also can be used at any step to enhance pain relief or counteract the adverse effects of medications.

Reprinted with permission from the American Academy of Hospice and Palliative Medicine. *Pocket Guide to Hospice/Palliative Medicine.*

PALLIATIVE AND END-OF-LIFE CARE: PAIN MANAGEMENT

WORLD HEALTH ORGANIZATION (WHO) ANALGESIC LADDER

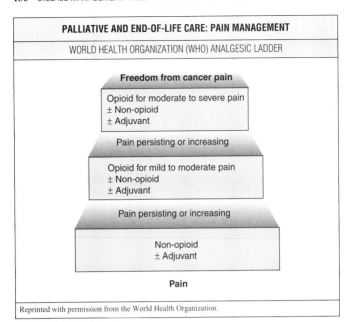

Freedom from cancer pain

Opioid for moderate to severe pain
± Non-opioid
± Adjuvant

Pain persisting or increasing

Opioid for mild to moderate pain
± Non-opioid
± Adjuvant

Pain persisting or increasing

Non-opioid
± Adjuvant

Pain

Reprinted with permission from the World Health Organization.

PAP SMEAR ABNORMALITIES: MANAGEMENT AND FOLLOW-UP[a]

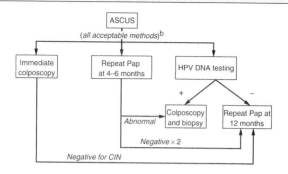

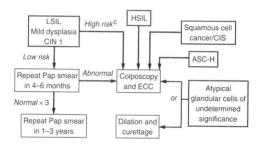

[a]Assumes satisfactory specimen; if unsatisfactory, repeat Pap smear. If no endocervical cells, follow-up in 1 year for low risk with previously negative smear, repeat in 4–6 mo. for high risk.

[b]Postmenopausal women: provide a course of intravaginal estrogen followed by repeat Pap smear 1 week after completing therapy. If repeat Pap negative, repeat in 4–6 months. If negative × 2, return to routine screening. If repeat test ASCUS or greater, refer for colposcopy. Immunosuppressed women should have immediate referral to colposcopy.

[c]High risk: history of abnormal Pap smear, high-risk HPV DNA, unlikely to return for follow-up.

ASCUS = atypical squamous cells of undetermined significance; ECC = endocervical curettage; LSIL = low-grade squamous intraepithelial lesion; CIN = cervical intraepithelial neoplasia; HSIL = high-grade squamous intraepithelial lesion; CIS = carcinoma in situ. ASC-H = atypical squamous cells, cannot exclude HSIL.

If endometrial cells are found in women aged ≥ 40 years, perform endometrial biopsy.

Source: Modified from JAMA 2002;287:2120–2129, Up-to-Date: Management of the abnormal Papanicolaou smear (www.uptodate.com, accessed 10/18/03).

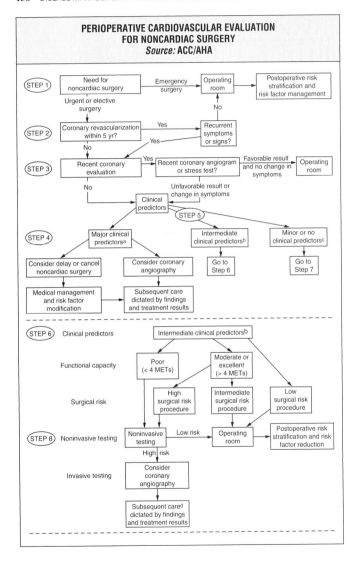

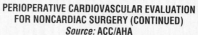

PERIOPERATIVE CARDIOVASCULAR EVALUATION FOR NONCARDIAC SURGERY (CONTINUED)
Source: ACC/AHA

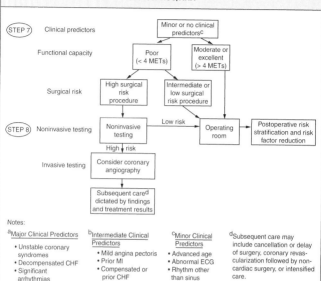

Notes:

^a**Major Clinical Predictors**
- Unstable coronary syndromes
- Decompensated CHF
- Significant arrhythmias
- Severe valvular disease

^b**Intermediate Clinical Predictors**
- Mild angina pectoris
- Prior MI
- Compensated or prior CHF
- Diabetes mellitus
- Renal insufficiency

^c**Minor Clinical Predictors**
- Advanced age
- Abnormal ECG
- Rhythm other than sinus
- Low functional capacity
- History of stroke
- Uncontrolled systemic hypertension

^dSubsequent care may include cancellation or delay of surgery, coronary revascularization followed by noncardiac surgery, or intensified care.

Source: Adapted from Eagle KA, Berger PB, Calkins H, et al. ACC/AHA guideline update for perioperative cardiovascular evaluation for noncardiac surgery update: a report of the American College of Cardiology/American Heart Association Task Force on Practice Guidelines (Committee to Update the 1996 Guidelines on Perioperative Cardiovascular Evaluation for Noncardiac Surgery). 2002. American College of Cardiology website. Available at: http://www.acc.org/clinical/guidelines/perio/update/periupdate_index.htm

COMMUNITY-ACQUIRED PNEUMONIA
Source: ATS

Group I	Group II	Group IIIa	Group IIIb
Outpatient No cardiopulm Hx[a] No modifying factors[b]	Outpatient w/ cardiopulm Hx[a] or modifiers[b]	Inpatients Not ICU No cardiopulm Hx[a] No modifying factors[b]	Inpatients Not ICU w/ cardiopulm Hx[a] or modifiers[b]
Azithromycin/ Clarithromycin or Doxycycline	Beta-Lactam *plus* Macrolide or doxycycline *OR* Fluoroquinolone[c]	IV azithromycin or Fluoroquinolone[c]	IV Beta-Lactam *plus* IV or oral macrolide or doxycycline *OR* Fluoroquinolone[c]

[a]Such as chronic obstructive pulmonary disease or congestive heart failure.

[b]Presence of risk factors for drug-resistant pneumococcus (aged > 65 yr, beta-lactam therapy within past 3 mo, alcoholism, immunosuppression, multiple medical comorbidities, exposure to child in day care center) presence of risk factors for gram-negative infection (residence in nursing home, cardiopulmonary disease, multiple medical comorbidities, recent antibiotic therapy), and risk factors for *Pseudomonas aeruginosa* [structural lung disease, corticosteroid therapy (>10 mg prednisone per day), broad spectrum antibiotic therapy for > 7 d past month, during malnutrition].

[c]Use fluoroquinolone with anti-streptococcus pneumonia activity.

Source: Modified from Am J Resp Crit Care Med 2001;163:1730–1754.

PRECONCEPTION GUIDELINES
Sources: ICSI and AAFP

Screening
  Abdominal/pelvic exam
  Blood pressure
  Breast exam
  Cholesterol, HDL
  Domestic abuse screening
  Height and weight
  Pap smear
  Risk profiles (infection, preterm labor, genetic disorders)
  Rubella/rubeola and varicella immunity (history, serology, or vaccination)

Counseling and education
  Accurate recording of menstrual dates
  Medications, supplements, vitamins
  Nutrition and weight
  Physical activity
  Preterm labor prevention
  Sexual practices
  Substance abuse
  Violence and abuse

Immunization and chemoprophylaxis
  Folate: 0.4–0.8 mg/day (4 mg/day if history of pregnancy with neural tube defect)
  Hepatitis B
  MMR
  Tetanus-diphtheria [Td] booster
  Varicella

Sources: Institute for Clinical Systems Improvement (ICSI). Routine prenatal care. Bloomington, MN: Institute for Clinical Systems Improvement, July 2003. AAFP. Summary of Policy Recommendations for Periodic Health Examinations, August 2003.

PRENATAL GUIDELINES Source: ICSI								
	Visit Timing (Weeks of Gestation)							
Item	**6–8**	**10–12**	**16–18**	**22**	**28**	**32**	**36**	**38–41**
ABO/Rh/Ab[a]	X				X			
Blood pressure		X	X	X	X	X	X	X
Body mechanics		X						
Breast feeding		X						
Check cervix					X		X	X
Chromosome/neural tube defect screening[b]		X	X					
Confirm fetal position							X	
Contraception							X	
Course of care	X							
Domestic violence	X				X			
Episiotomy						X		
Fetal growth		X			X			
Fetal heart tones		X	X	X	X	X	X	X
Fetal movement					X			
Fundal height			X	X	X	X	X	X
Gestational DM[c]					X			
Group B strep culture							X	
Height	X							
Hepatitis Bs Ag	X							
Hemoglobin	X							
HIV[d]	X							
Infant CPR								X
Infectious disease risk[e]					X			
Influenza					X			

PRENATAL GUIDELINES (CONTINUED) *Source:* ICSI								
	Visit Timing (Weeks of Gestation)							
Item	**6–8**	**10–12**	**16–18**	**22**	**28**	**32**	**36**	**38–41**
Labor and delivery						X		X
Late pregnancy symptoms							X	
Nutrition	X							
Nutritional supplements	X							
OB H&P	X							
OB ultrasound (optional)			X					
Pediatric care[f]						X		
Physiology of pregnancy	X		X		X			
Postpartum care							X	X
Preregistration					X			
Preterm labor risk					X			
Preterm labor symptoms				X	X			
Rh antibody status					X			
Quickening			X					
Risk profiles[g]	X							
RPR[h]	X							
Rubella/rubeola	X							
Second trimester growth			X					
Sexuality						X		
Td booster	X							
Travel						X		
Triple screen			X					
Urine culture	X							

PRENATAL GUIDELINES (CONTINUED)
Source: ICSI

Item	6–8	10–12	16–18	22	28	32	36	38–41
	visit timing							

Item	Visit Timing (Weeks of Gestation)							
	6–8	10–12	16–18	22	28	32	36	38–41
Varicella	X							
Warning signs	X					X		
Weight	X	X	X	X	X	X	X	X
When to call							X	
Work					X			

[a]**USPSTF** strongly recommends Rh (D) blood typing and antibody testing for all pregnant women during their first visit for pregnancy-related care. Repeat Rh (D) antibody testing is recommended for all unsensitized Rh (D)–negative women at 24–28 weeks' gestation, unless the biological father is known to be Rh (D) negative.

[b]Maternal serum triple screen, alpha-fetoprotein (AFP), human chorionic gonadotropin (HCG), and estriol, is performed optimally at 16 weeks. Alternatives to the triple screen are emerging. Nuchal translucency (NT) and first-trimester serum screening are available on a limited basis.

[c]**AAFP:** Evidence insufficient to recommend for or against routine screening for gestational diabetes in asymptomatic pregnant women. Fourth International Workshop-Conference on Gestational Diabetes Mellitus (GDM) [Diabetes Care 2004;27(Suppl 1):S88–S90]: Risk assessment for GDM at the first prenatal visit. If high risk of GDM (marked obesity, personal history of GDM, glycosuria, strong family history of DM), undergo glucose testing as soon as feasible. If normal, retest at 24–28 weeks' gestation. If average risk, undergo glucose testing at 24–28 weeks' gestation. If low risk (age < 25 years, prepregnancy weight normal, ethnic group with low prevalence of GDM, no known DM in first-degree relatives, no history of abnormal glucose tolerance, no history of poor obstetric outcome), no glucose testing. **USPSTF:** Could not determine the balance of benefits and harms of screening for GDM. [Obstet Gynecol 2003;101(2):393–395]

[d]**U.S. Public Health Service:** HIV screening should be a routine part of prenatal care for all women. HIV testing should be voluntary and free of coercion. [MMWR Recomm Rep 2001;50(RR-19):59–86]

[e]**AAFP** recommends screening all asymptomatic pregnant females aged 25 years or younger for chlamydia. AAFP recommends screening pregnant women at high risk for gonorrhea (new or multiple sexual partners in the past 12 months; presence of other sexually transmitted infections, including HIV; and sexual contacts of persons with gonorrhea or chlamydia).

[f]**AAP** recommends five objectives for prenatal pediatrician visit: 1) establishing the relationship between physician and parents, 2) gathering basic information, 3) providing information and advice, 4) building parenting skills, and 5) identifying high-risk situations. [Pediatrics 2001;107(6):1456–1458]

[g]Assess for risk of or related to preterm labor, workplace hazards, lifestyle, infectious disease, genetics.

[h]**AAFP** strongly recommends screening for syphilis in pregnant women.

Source: Institute for Clinical Systems Improvement (ICSI). Routine prenatal care. Bloomington, MN: Institute for Clinical Systems Improvement (ICSI), July 2003.

PERI- AND POSTNATAL GUIDELINES *Sources:* AAFP 2003 and Pediatrics 2004;114:297–316	
Breastfeeding	Strongly recommends counseling to promote breastfeeding through at least 6 months of age.
Hearing loss, sensorineural	Insufficient evidence for or against routine screening of newborns for hearing loss during the postpartum hospitalization period.
Hemoglobinopathies	Strongly recommends ordering screening tests for hemoglobinopathies in neonates.
Hyperbilirubinemia	Perform ongoing systematic assessments during the neonatal period for the risk of an infant developing severe hyperbilirubinemia.
Phenylketonuria	Strongly recommends ordering screening tests for phenylketonuria in neonates.
Thyroid function abnormalities	Strongly recommends ordering screening tests for thyroid function abnormalities in neonates.

TOBACCO CESSATION TREATMENT ALGORITHM
Source: U.S. Public Health Service

Five A's

1. Ask about tobacco use.

2. Advise to quit through clear personalized messages.

3. Assess willingness to quit.

4. Assist to quit,[a] including referral to Quit Lines (e.g., 1-800-NO-BUTTS).

5. Arrange follow-up and support.

[a]Physicians can assist patients to quit by devising a quit plan, providing problem-solving counseling, providing intratreatment social support, helping patients obtain social support from their environment/friends, and recommending pharmacotherapy for appropriate patients. Use caution in recommending pharmacotherapy in patients with medical contraindications, those smoking < 10 cigarettes per day, pregnant/breastfeeding women, and adolescent smokers.
Source: Fiore MC et al. Treating Tobacco Use and Dependence. Quick Reference Guide for Clinicians. Rockville, MD: U.S. Department of Health and Human Services. Public Health Service, October 2000.

MOTIVATING TOBACCO USERS TO QUIT

Five R's

1. Relevance: personal

2. Risks: Acute, long-term, environmental

3. Rewards: have patient identify (e.g., save money, better food taste)

4. Road blocks: help problem-solve

5. Repetition: at every office visit

| | TOBACCO CESSATION TREATMENT OPTIONS | | | | | |

TOBACCO CESSATION TREATMENT OPTIONS[a]

Pharmacotherapy	Precautions/ Contraindications	Side Effects	Dosage	Duration	Availability	Cost/Day[b]
First-line pharmacotherapies (approved for use for smoking cessation by the FDA)						
Bupropion SR	History of seizure History of eating disorder	Insomnia Dry mouth	150 mg every morning for 3 days, then 150 mg twice daily. (Begin treatment 1–2 weeks pre-quit.)	7–12 weeks maintenance up to 6 months	Zyban (prescription only)	$3.33
Nicotine gum	—	Mouth soreness Dyspepsia	1–24 cigs/day: 2-mg gum (up to 24 pieces/day). 25+ cigs/day: 4-mg gum (up to 24 pieces/day).	Up to 12 weeks	Nicorette, Nicorette Mint (OTC only)	$6.25 for 10 2-mg pieces $6.87 for 10 4-mg pieces
Nicotine inhaler	—	Local irritation of mouth and throat	6–16 cartridges/day	Up to 6 months	Nicotrol Inhaler (prescription only)	$10.94 for 10 cartridges
Nicotine nasal spray	—	Nasal irritation	8–40 doses/day	3–6 months	Nicotrol NS (prescription only)	$5.40 for 12 doses
Nicotine patch	—	Local skin reaction Insomnia	21 mg/24 hours 14 mg/24 hours 7 mg/24 hours 15 mg/16 hours	4 weeks Then 2 weeks Then 2 weeks 8 weeks	Nicoderm CQ (OTC only), Generic patches (prescription and OTC) Nicotrol (OTC only)	Brand-name patches $4.00–$4.50[c]

TOBACCO CESSATION TREATMENT OPTIONS[a] (CONTINUED)

Second-line pharmacotherapies (not approved for use for smoking cessation by the FDA)

Pharmacotherapy	Precautions/ Contraindications	Side Effects	Dosage	Duration	Availability	Cost/Day[b]
Clonidine	Rebound hypertension	Dry mouth Drowsiness Dizziness Sedation	0.15–0.75 mg/day	3–10 weeks	Oral Clonidine-generic (prescription only), Catapres (prescription only), Transdermal Catapres (prescription only)	Clonidine $0.24 for 0.2 mg; Catapres (transdermal) $3.50
Nortriptyline	Risk of arrhythmias	Sedation Dry mouth	75–100 mg/day	12 weeks	Nortriptyline HCl-generic (prescription only)	$0.74 for 75 mg

[a]The information contained within this table is not comprehensive. Please see package insert for additional information.
[b]Prices based on retail prices of medication purchased at a national chain pharmacy, located in Madison, WI, April 2000.
[c]Generic brands of the patch recently became available and may be less expensive.
Source: U.S. Public Health Service.

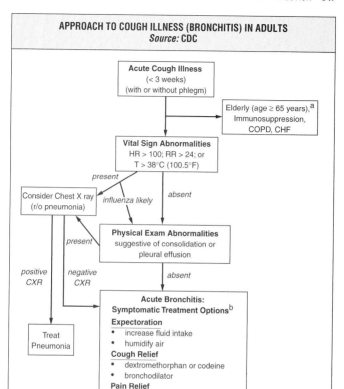

APPROACH TO COUGH ILLNESS (BRONCHITIS) IN ADULTS
Source: CDC

[a]Pneumonia in the elderly, as well as those with comorbidity, often presents atypically. Evaluation should be individualized.

[b]If duration of illness is > 2 weeks, consider pertussis. PCR or culture testing for pertussis is done to confirm the diagnosis and indicate the need for public health follow-up to prevent illness among contacts, especially infants. Antibiotic therapy can decrease shedding, but has no effect on symptoms during the paroxysmal phase (≥ 10 days after illness onset). Treat with erythromycin × 14 days pending results.

Source: Adapted from Centers for Disease Control and Prevention; Ann Intern Med 2001; 134:521.

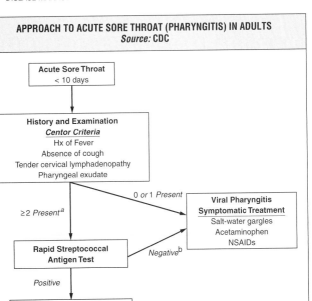

APPROACH TO ACUTE SORE THROAT (PHARYNGITIS) IN ADULTS
Source: CDC

Acute Sore Throat
< 10 days

History and Examination
Centor Criteria
Hx of Fever
Absence of cough
Tender cervical lymphadenopathy
Pharyngeal exudate

0 or 1 *Present*

≥2 *Present*[a]

Rapid Streptococcal
Antigen Test

Negative[b]

Viral Pharyngitis
Symptomatic Treatment
Salt-water gargles
Acetaminophen
NSAIDs

Positive

**Streptococcal Pharyngitis
Antibiotic Treatment**
Penicillin or erythromycin
(penicillin allergic); as well as
symptomatic treatment

[a]Acceptable alternatives to these strategies include: 1) test and treat patients with 2 or 3 Centor criteria present, and empirically treat with antibiotics (do not test) patients with 4 Centor criteria; or 2) do not test any patients, and empirically treat with antibiotics patients with 3 or 4 Centor criteria present.

[b]Do not recommend culture-confirmation of negative rapid antigen tests in adults when the sensitivity of the rapid antigen test exceeds 80%. When performed in adults with ≥ 2 criteria present, the sensitivity exceeds 90%. (Ann Emerg Med 2001;38:648)

These principles apply to immunocompetent adults without complicated comorbidities such as chronic lung or heart disease, history of rheumatic fever, or during known group A streptococcal outbreaks. They also are not intended to apply during a known epidemic of acute rheumatic fever or streptococcal pharyngitis, or for nonindustrialized countries where the endemic rate of acute rheumatic fever is much higher than it is in the U.S.

Source: Adapted from Centers for Disease Control and Prevention; Ann Intern Med 2001; 134:509.

APPROACH TO ACUTE NASAL AND SINUS CONGESTION (SINUSITIS) IN ADULTS
Source: CDC

**Acute Rhinosinusitis
(< 4 weeks duration)**
Stuffy nose
Nasal discharge
Facial pressure

Symptomatic Therapy
Nasal saline lavage
Decongestants (nasal and/or oral)
NSAIDs and acetaminophen
Antihistamines (if allergic component)

< 7 day duration *≥ 7 day duration* *Any duration*

Uncomplicated Rhinosinusitis
• Symptomatic therapy only

**Bacterial Rhinosinusitis
Risk Factors**
• Purulent nasal discharge
  PLUS
• Facial pain or tenderness,
  or tooth pain or tenderness

Acute Focal Sinusitis
Acute toxic presentation:
• severe facial pain or
  toothache
• unilateral redness and/
  or edema
• fever (oral temp > 38°C)

present

Antibiotic Therapy
• Consider amoxicillin for
  mild to moderate cases.
  Acute focal sinusitis should
  be treated in consultation with
  ENT or infectious disease
  experts (may require urgent
  drainage).

The above principles apply to the diagnosis and treatment of acute maxillary and ethmoid rhinosinusitis in non-immunocompromised adults.

Source: Adapted from Centers for Disease Control and Prevention; Ann Intern Med 2001; 134:498.

UTI IN WOMEN: DIAGNOSIS AND MANAGEMENT
Source: University of Michigan Health System

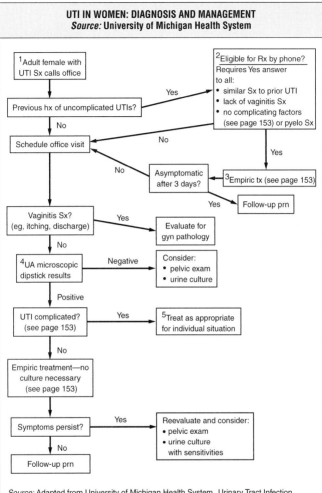

Source: Adapted from University of Michigan Health System, Urinary Tract Infection guideline, June 1999; Infectious Diseases Society of America (IDSA) practice guideline (Clinical Infectious Diseases 1999;29:745–758); Am J Med 1999;106:636–641; NEJM 2003;349:259–266.

UTI IN WOMEN ALGORITHM, NOTES AND TABLES

LABORATORY CHARGES AND RELATIVE COSTS

Test	Relative Cost
Urinalysis, dipstick	$
Urinalysis, complete microscopic	$$
Urine culture	$$$

COMPLICATING FACTORS

Catheter

Diabetes mellitus

Immunosuppression

Nephrolithiasis

Pregnancy

Pyelonephritis symptoms

Recent hospitalization or nursing home residence

Recurrent UTIs (3/year)

Symptoms for > 7 days

Urologic structural/functional abnormality

TREATMENT REGIMENS AND RELATIVE COSTS

Treatment Regimen	Relative Cost
First Line	
Trimethoprim/Sulfa DS BID × 3 days	$
Second Line (in preferred order)	
Trimethoprim 100 mg TID × 3 days	$
Ciprofloxacin 100 mg BID × 3 days	$$
Norfloxacin 400 mg BID × 3 days	$$$
Ofloxacin 200 mg BID × 3 days	$$$
Amoxicillin 500 mg TID × 7 days	$$
Nitrofurantoin 100 mg QID × 7 days	$$$$
Nitrofurantoin 100 mg BID × 7 days	$$$

1. The majority of UTIs occur in sexually active women. Risk increases by 3–5 times when diaphragms are used for contraception. Risk also increases slightly with not voiding after sexual intercourse and use of spermicides. Dysuria with either urgency or frequency, in the absence of vaginal symptoms, yields a prior probability of UTI of 70%–80%. Generally, UTI symptoms are of abrupt onset (< 3 days).

2. The majority of UTIs in women are uncomplicated and resolve readily with brief courses of antibiotics. Therefore, many women can be assessed and safely managed without an office visit or laboratory examination. A study of a telephone-based clinical practice guideline for managing presumed uncomplicated cystitis among women aged 18–55 years found that guideline implementation significantly decreased the proportion of patients with presumed cystitis who received urinalysis, urine culture, or an initial office visit. The guideline also increased the proportion of women who received a guideline-recommended antibiotic. Adverse outcomes (return office visit, sexually transmitted disease, pyelonephritis within 60 days of initial diagnosis) did not increase as a result of guideline implementation. The study authors concluded that guideline use decreased laboratory utilization and overall costs while maintaining or improving the quality of care for patients who were presumptively treated for acute uncomplicated cystitis. (Saint S, Scholes D, Fihn S, Farrell R, Stamm W. The effectiveness of a clinical practice guideline for the management of presumed uncomplicated urinary tract infection in women. Am J Med 1999;106:636–641)

3. Acute uncomplicated cystitis in women traditionally has been treated with longer (7–10 day) courses of antibiotics. More recent studies have found shorter courses (3–5 days) of oral antibiotics to be as effective as traditional courses. A review of 28 treatment trials of adult women with uncomplicated cystitis concluded that no benefit was achieved by increasing the length of therapy beyond 5 days. (Norrby SR. Short-term treatment of uncomplicated lower urinary tract infections in women. Rev Infect Dis 1990;12:458–467) The optimal treatment of uncomplicated UTI in patients who are not allergic or sensitive is 3 days of TMP/SMX.

4. *Dipstick analysis* for leukocyte esterase, an indirect test for the presence for pyuria, is the least expensive and least time-intensive diagnostic test for UTI. It is estimated to have a sensitivity of 75%–96% and specificity of 94%–98%. Nitrite testing by dipstick is less useful, in large part because it is only positive in the presence of bacteria that produce nitrate reductase, and can be confounded by consumption of ascorbic acid. *Microscopic examination* of unstained, centrifuged urine by a trained observer under 40 × power has a sensitivity of 82%–97% and a specificity of 84%–95%. For urine culture, sensitivity varies from 50%–95%, depending on the threshold for UTI, and specificity varies from 85%–99%. Because of the limited sensitivity of urine culture, and the delay required for results, urine culture is not recommended to diagnose or verify uncomplicated UTI.

5. Unlike women with uncomplicated UTI, care for women with complicating factors includes:

- *Culture:* Obtain pretreatment culture and sensitivity.
- *Treatment:* Initiate treatment with trimethoprim/sulfa or quinolone for 7–14 days (quinolones contraindicated in pregnancy).
- *Follow-up UA:* Obtain follow-up urinalysis to document clearing.
- *Possible structural evaluation:* Lower threshold for urologic structural evaluation with cysto/IVP.

4
Appendices

SCREENING INSTRUMENTS: ALCOHOL ABUSE

SENSITIVITY AND SPECIFICITY OF SCREENING TESTS FOR PROBLEM DRINKING

Instrument Name	Screening Questions/Scoring	Threshold Score	Sensitivity/Specificity (%)	Source
CAGE[a]	See page 157	> 1 > 2 > 3	77/58 53/81 29/92	Am J Psychiatr 1974;131:1121 J Gen Intern Med 1998;13:379
AUDIT	See page 157	> 4 > 5 > 6	87/70 77/84 66/90	BMJ 1997;314:420 J Gen Intern Med 1998;13:379

[a]The CAGE may be less applicable to binge drinkers (eg, college students), the elderly, and minority populations.

SCREENING INSTRUMENTS: ALCOHOL ABUSE

SCREENING PROCEDURES FOR PROBLEM DRINKING

1. CAGE screening test[a]

Have you ever felt the need to **C**ut down on drinking?

Have you ever felt **A**nnoyed by criticism of your drinking?

Have you ever felt **G**uilty about your drinking?

Have you ever taken a morning **E**ye opener?

INTERPRETATION: Two "yes" answers are considered a positive screen. One "yes" answer should arouse a suspicion of alcohol abuse.

2. The Alcohol Use Disorder Identification Test (AUDIT).[b] (Scores for response categories are given in parentheses. Scores range from 0 to 40, with a cutoff score of ≥ 5 indicating hazardous drinking, harmful drinking, or alcohol dependence.)

1) How often do you have a drink containing alcohol?

(0) Never   (1) Monthly or less   (2) Two to four times a month   (3) Two or three times a week   (4) Four or more times a week

2) How many drinks containing alcohol do you have on a typical day when you are drinking?

(0) 1 or 2   (1) 3 or 4   (2) 5 or 6   (3) 7 to 9   (4) 10 or more

3) How often do you have six or more drinks on one occasion?

(0) Never   (1) Less than monthly   (2) Monthly   (3) Weekly   (4) Daily or almost daily

4) How often during the past year have you found that you were not able to stop drinking once you had started?

(0) Never   (1) Less than monthly   (2) Monthly   (3) Weekly   (4) Daily or almost daily

5) How often during the past year have you failed to do what was normally expected of you because of drinking?

(0) Never   (1) Less than monthly   (2) Monthly   (3) Weekly   (4) Daily or almost daily

SCREENING INSTRUMENTS: ALCOHOL ABUSE

SCREENING PROCEDURES FOR PROBLEM DRINKING (CONTINUED)

6) How often during the past year have you needed a first drink in the morning to get yourself going after a heavy drinking session?

(0) Never   (1) Less than monthly   (2) Monthly   (3) Weekly   (4) Daily or almost daily

7) How often during the past year have you had a feeling of guilt or remorse after drinking?

(0) Never   (1) Less than monthly   (2) Monthly   (3) Weekly   (4) Daily or almost daily

8) How often during the past year have you been unable to remember what happened the night before because you had been drinking?

(0) Never   (1) Less than monthly   (2) Monthly   (3) Weekly   (4) Daily or almost daily

9) Have you or has someone else been injured as a result of your drinking?

(0) No   (2) Yes, but not in the past year   (4) Yes, during the past year

10) Has a relative or friend or a doctor or other health worker been concerned about your drinking or suggested you cut down?

(0) No   (2) Yes, but not in the past year   (4) Yes, during the past year

[a]Modified from Mayfield D et al. The CAGE questionnaire: Validation of a new alcoholism screening instrument. Am J Psychiatry 1974;131:1121.
[b]From Piccinelli M et al. Efficacy of the alcohol use disorders identification test as a screening tool for hazardous alcohol intake and related disorders in primary care: A validity study. BMJ 1997;314:420.

SCREENING INSTRUMENTS: COGNITIVE IMPAIRMENT

THE ANNOTATED MINI MENTAL STATE EXAMINATION (AMMSE)

MiniMental LLC

Suspect dementia
when score ≤ 24.

NAME OF SUBJECT _____ Age _____

NAME OF EXAMINER _____ Years of School Completed ____

Approach the patient with respect and encouragement. Date of Examination _____

Ask: Do you have any trouble with your memory? ☐ Yes ☐ No

May I ask you some questions about your memory? ☐ Yes ☐ No

SCORE ITEM

5 ( ) **TIME ORIENTATION**
Ask:
What is the year _____ (1), season _____ (1),
month of the year _____ (1), date _____ (1),
day of the week _____ (1)?

5 ( ) **PLACE ORIENTATION**
Ask:
Where are we now? What is the state _____ (1), city _____ (1),
part of the city_____ (1), building _____ (1),
floor of the building _____ (1)?

3 ( ) **REGISTRATION OF THREE WORDS**
Say: Listen carefully. I am going to say three words. You say them back after I stop.
Ready? Here they are...PONY (wait 1 second), QUARTER (wait 1 second), ORANGE
(wait 1 second). What were those words?
_____ (1)
_____ (1)
_____ (1)
Give 1 point for each correct answer, then repeat them until the patient learns all three.

5 ( ) **SERIAL 7s AS A TEST OF ATTENTION AND CALCULATION**
Ask: Subtract 7 from 100 and continue to subtract 7 from each subsequent remainder
until I tell you to stop. What is 100 take away 7?_____ (1)
Say:
Keep going. _____ (1), _____ (1),
_____ (1), _____ (1).

3 ( ) **RECALL OF THREE WORDS**
Ask:
What were those three words I asked you to remember?
Give one point for each correct answer. _____ (1),
_____ (1), _____ (1).

2 ( ) **NAMING**
Ask:
What is this? (show pencil) _____ (1). What is this? (show watch) _____ (1).

For more
information or
additional copies
of this exam,
call (617)587-4215

© 1975, 1998 MiniMental LLC

SCREENING INSTRUMENTS:
COGNITIVE IMPAIRMENT (CONTINUED)

MiniMental LLC

1 ( ) **REPETITION**
Say:
Now I am going to ask you to repeat what I say. Ready? No ifs, ands or buts.
Now you say that. _____ (1)

3 ( ) **COMPREHENSION**
Say:
Listen carefully because I am going to ask you to do something.
Take this paper in your left hand (1), fold it in half (1), and put it on the floor. (1)

1 ( ) **READING**
Say:
Please read the following and do what it says, but do not say it aloud. (1)

Close your eyes

1 ( ) **WRITING**
Say:
Please write a sentence. If the patient does not respond, say: Write about the weather. (1)

_____

_____

1 ( ) **DRAWING**
Say: Please copy this design.

TOTAL SCORE _____ Assess level of consciousness along a continuum

Alert	Drowsy	Stupor	Coma

	YES NO		YES NO	FUNCTION BY PROXY

Cooperative: ☐ ☐   Deterioration from   Please record date when patient was last able to perform the following tasks.
Depressed: ☐ ☐   previous level of   Ask caregiver if patient independently handles:
Anxious: ☐ ☐   functioning: ☐ ☐
Poor Vision: ☐ ☐   Family History of Dementia: ☐ ☐   YES NO DATE
Poor Hearing: ☐ ☐   Head Trauma: ☐ ☐   Money/Bills: ☐ ☐ ____
Native Language: Stroke: ☐ ☐   Medication: ☐ ☐ ____
_____   Alcohol Abuse: ☐ ☐   Transportation: ☐ ☐ ____
                Thyroid Disease: ☐ ☐   Telephone: ☐ ☐ ____

SCREENING INSTRUMENTS: DEPRESSION

SCREENING TESTS FOR DEPRESSION

Instrument Name	Screening Questions/Scoring	Threshold Score	Source
Beck Depression Inventory (Short Form)	See page 162	0–4: None or minimal depression 5–7: Mild depression 8–15: Moderate depression > 15: Severe depression	Postgrad Med 1972;Dec:81
Geriatric Depression Scale	See page 163	≥ 15: Depression	J Psychiatr Res 1983;17:37
PRIME-MD© (mood questions)	(1) During the past month, have you often been bothered by feeling down, depressed, or hopeless? (2) During the past month, have you often been bothered by little interest or pleasure in doing things?	"Yes" to either question[a]	JAMA 1994;272:1749 J Gen Intern Med 1997;12:439

[a]Sensitivity 86%–96%; specificity 57%–75%.
©Pfizer Inc.

SCREENING INSTRUMENTS: DEPRESSION

BECK DEPRESSION INVENTORY, SHORT FORM

Instructions: This is a questionnaire. On the questionnaire are groups of statements. Please read the entire group of statements in each category. Then pick out the one statement in that group that best describes the way you feel today, that is, *right now!* Circle the number beside the statement you have chosen. If several statements in the group seem to apply equally well, circle each one. Sum all numbers to calculate a score.

Be sure to read all the statements in each group before making your choice.

A. Sadness
3 I am so sad or unhappy that I can't stand it.
2 I am blue or sad all the time and I can't snap out of it.
1 I feel sad or blue.
0 I do not feel sad.

B. Pessimism
3 I feel that the future is hopeless and that things cannot improve.
2 I feel I have nothing to look forward to.
1 I feel discouraged about the future.
0 I am not particularly pessimistic or discouraged about the future.

C. Sense of failure
3 I feel I am a complete failure as a person (parent, husband, wife).
2 As I look back on my life, all I can see is a lot of failures.
1 I feel I have failed more than the average person.
0 I do not feel like a failure.

D. Dissatisfaction
3 I am dissatisfied with everything.
2 I don't get satisfaction out of anything anymore.
1 I don't enjoy things the way I used to.
0 I am not particularly dissatisfied.

E. Guilt
3 I feel as though I am very bad or worthless.
2 I feel quite guilty.
1 I feel bad or unworthy a good part of the time.
0 I don't feel particularly guilty.

F. Self-dislike
3 I hate myself.
2 I am disgusted with myself.
1 I am disappointed in myself.
0 I don't feel disappointed in myself.

G. Self-harm
3 I would kill myself if I had the chance.
2 I have definite plans about committing suicide.
1 I feel I would be better off dead.
0 I don't have any thoughts of harming myself.

H. Social withdrawal
3 I have lost all of my interest in other people and don't care about them at all.
2 I have lost most of my interest in other people and have little feeling for them.
1 I am less interested in other people than I used to be.
0 I have not lost interest in other people.

I. Indecisiveness
3 I can't make any decisions at all anymore.
2 I have great difficulty in making decisions.
1 I try to put off making decisions.
0 I make decisions about as well as ever.

J. Self-image change
3 I feel that I am ugly or repulsive-looking.
2 I feel that there are permanent changes in my appearance and they make me look unattractive.
1 I am worried that I am looking old or unattractive.
0 I don't feel that I look any worse than I used to.

SCREENING INSTRUMENTS: DEPRESSION

BECK DEPRESSION INVENTORY, SHORT FORM (CONTINUED)

K. Work difficulty
3 I can't do any work at all.
2 I have to push myself very hard to do anything.
1 It takes extra effort to get started at doing something.
0 I can work about as well as before.

L. Fatigability
3 I get too tired to do anything.

2 I get tired from doing anything.
1 I get tired more easily than I used to.
0 I don't get any more tired than usual.

M. Anorexia
3 I have no appetite at all anymore.
2 My appetite is much worse now.
1 My appetite is not as good as it used to be.
0 My appetite is no worse than usual.

Source: Reproduced with permission from Beck AT, Beck RW. Screening depressed patients in family practice: A rapid technic. Postgrad Med 1972;52:81.

GERIATRIC DEPRESSION SCALE

Choose the best answer for how you felt over the past week

1. Are you basically satisfied with your life? yes / no
2. Have you dropped many of your activities and interests? yes / no
3. Do you feel that your life is empty? yes / no
4. Do you often get bored? yes / no
5. Are you hopeful about the future? yes / no
6. Are you bothered by thoughts you can't get out of your head? yes / no
7. Are you in good spirits most of the time? yes / no
8. Are you afraid that something bad is going to happen to you? yes / no
9. Do you feel happy most of the time? yes / no
10. Do you often feel helpless? yes / no
11. Do you often get restless and fidgety? yes / no
12. Do you prefer to stay at home, rather than going out and doing new things? yes / no
13. Do you frequently worry about the future? yes / no
14. Do you feel you have more problems with memory than most? yes / no
15. Do you think it is wonderful to be alive now? yes / no
16. Do you often feel downhearted and blue? yes / no
17. Do you feel pretty worthless the way you are now? yes / no
18. Do you worry a lot about the past? yes / no
19. Do you find life very exciting? yes / no
20. Is it hard for you to get started on new projects? yes / no
21. Do you feel full of energy? yes / no
22. Do you feel that your situation is hopeless? yes / no
23. Do you think that most people are better off than you are? yes / no

SCREENING INSTRUMENTS: DEPRESSION	
GERIATRIC DEPRESSION SCALE	
Choose the best answer for how you felt over the past week	
24. Do you frequently get upset over little things?	yes / no
25. Do you frequently feel like crying?	yes / no
26. Do you have trouble concentrating?	yes / no
27. Do you enjoy getting up in the morning?	yes / no
28. Do you prefer to avoid social gatherings?	yes / no
29. Is it easy for you to make decisions?	yes / no
30. Is your mind as clear as it used to be?	yes / no

One point for each response suggestive of depression. (Specifically "no" responses to questions 1, 5, 7, 9, 15, 19, 21, 27, 29, and 30, and "yes" responses to the remaining questions are suggestive of depression.)

A score of ≥ 15 yields a sensitivity of 80% and a specificity of 100%, as a screening test for geriatric depression. Clin Gerontologist 1982;1:37.

Source: Reproduced with permission from Yesavage JA et al. Development and validation of a geriatric depression screening scale: A preliminary report. J Psychiatr Res 1982–83;17:37

FUNCTIONAL ASSESSMENT SCREENING IN THE ELDERLY

Target Area	Assessment Procedure	Abnormal Result	Suggested Intervention
Vision	Ask: "Do you have difficulty driving or watching television or reading or doing any of your daily activities because of your eyesight?" Test each eye with Jaeger card while patient wears corrective lenses (if applicable).	"Yes" and inability to read greater than 20/40	Refer to ophthalmologist.
Hearing	Whisper a short, easily answered question such as "What is your name?" in each ear while the examiner's face is out of direct view. Use audioscope set at 40 dB; test using 1,000 and 2,000 Hz.	Inability to answer question Inability to hear 1,000 or 2,000 Hz in both ears or inability to hear frequencies in either ear	Examine auditory canals for cerumen and clean if necessary. Repeat test; if still abnormal in either ear, refer for audiometry and possible prosthesis.
Arm	Proximal: "Touch the back of your head with both hands." Distal: "Pick up the spoon."	Inability to do task	Examine the arm fully (muscle, joint, and nerve), paying attention to pain, weakness, limited range of motion. Consider referral for physical therapy.
Leg	Observe the patient after instructing as follows: "Rise from your chair, walk 10 feet, return, and sit down."	Inability to complete task in 15 seconds	Do full neurologic and musculoskeletal evaluation, paying attention to strength, pain, range of motion, balance, and gait. Consider referral for physical therapy.
Continence of urine	Ask, "Do you ever lose your urine and get wet?" If yes, then ask, "Have you lost urine on at least 6 separate days?"	"Yes" to both questions	Ascertain frequency and amount. Search for remediable causes, including local irritations, polyuric states, and medications. Consider urologic referral.

FUNCTIONAL ASSESSMENT SCREENING IN THE ELDERLY (CONTINUED)			
Target Area	**Assessment Procedure**	**Abnormal Result**	**Suggested Intervention**
Nutrition	Ask, "Without trying, have you lost 10 lb or more in the last 6 months?" Weigh the patient. Measure height.	"Yes" or weight is below acceptable range for height	Do appropriate medical evaluation.
Mental status	Instruct as follows: "I am going to name three objects (pencil, truck, book). I will ask you to repeat their names now and then again a few minutes from now."	Inability to recall all three objects after 1 minute	Administer Folstein Mini-Mental State Examination. If score is less than 24, search for causes of cognitive impairment. Ascertain onset, duration, and fluctuation of overt symptoms. Review medications. Assess consciousness and affect. Do appropriate laboratory tests.
Depression	Ask, "Do you often feel sad or depressed?" or "How are your spirits?"	"Yes" or "Not very good, I guess"	Administer Geriatric Depression Scale. If positive (score above 15), check for antihypertensive, psychotropic, or other pertinent medications. Consider appropriate pharmacologic or psychiatric treatment.
ADL-IADL[a]	Ask, "Can you get out of bed yourself?" "Can you dress yourself?" "Can you make your own meals?" "Can you do your own shopping?"	"No" to any question	Corroborate responses with patient's appearance; question family members if accuracy is uncertain. Determine reasons for the inability (motivation compared with physical limitation). Institute appropriate medical, social, or environmental interventions.

FUNCTIONAL ASSESSMENT SCREENING IN THE ELDERLY (CONTINUED)

Target Area	Assessment Procedure	Abnormal Result	Suggested Intervention
Home environment	Ask, "Do you have trouble with stairs inside or outside of your home?" Ask about potential hazards inside the home with bathtubs, rugs, or lighting.	"Yes"	Evaluate home safety and institute appropriate countermeasures.
Social support	Ask, "Who would be able to help you in case of illness or emergency?"	—	List identified persons in the medical record. Become familiar with available resources for the elderly in the community.

[a]Activities of Daily Living–Instrumental Activities of Daily Living.
Source: Modified from Lachs MS et al. A simple procedure for screening for functional disability in elderly patients. Ann Intern Med 1990;112:699.
Geriatrics at your fingertips online edition 2004 (http://www.geriatricsatyourfingertips.org, accessed 7/23/04).

95TH PERCENTILE OF BLOOD PRESSURE FOR BOYS

Age (y)	SBP (mm Hg) by percentile of height							DBP (mm Hg) by percentile of height						
	5%	10%	25%	50%	75%	90%	95%	5%	10%	25%	50%	75%	90%	95%
3	104	105	107	109	110	112	113	63	63	64	65	66	67	67
4	106	107	109	111	112	114	115	66	67	68	69	70	71	71
5	108	109	110	112	114	115	116	69	70	71	72	73	74	74
6	109	110	112	114	115	117	117	72	72	73	74	75	76	76
7	110	111	113	115	117	118	119	74	74	75	76	77	78	78
8	111	112	114	116	118	119	120	75	76	77	78	79	79	80
9	113	114	116	118	119	121	121	76	77	78	79	80	81	81
10	115	116	117	119	121	122	123	77	78	79	80	81	81	82
11	117	118	119	121	123	124	125	78	78	79	80	81	82	82
12	119	120	122	123	125	127	127	78	79	80	81	82	82	83
13	121	122	124	126	128	129	130	79	79	80	81	82	83	83
14	124	125	127	128	130	132	132	80	80	81	82	83	84	84
15	126	127	129	131	133	134	135	81	81	82	83	84	85	85
16	129	130	132	134	135	137	137	82	83	83	84	85	86	87
17	131	132	134	136	138	139	140	84	85	86	87	87	88	89

95TH PERCENTILE OF BLOOD PRESSURE FOR GIRLS

Age (y)	SBP (mm Hg) by percentile of height							DBP (mm Hg) by percentile of height						
	5%	10%	25%	50%	75%	90%	95%	5%	10%	25%	50%	75%	90%	95%
3	104	104	105	107	108	109	110	65	66	66	67	68	68	69
4	105	106	107	108	110	111	112	68	68	69	70	71	71	72
5	107	107	108	110	111	112	113	70	71	71	72	73	73	74
6	108	109	110	111	113	114	115	72	72	73	74	74	75	76
7	110	111	112	113	115	116	116	73	74	74	75	76	76	77
8	112	112	114	115	116	118	118	75	75	75	76	77	78	78
9	114	114	115	117	118	119	120	76	76	76	77	78	79	79
10	116	116	117	119	120	121	122	77	77	78	78	79	80	80
11	118	118	119	121	122	123	124	78	78	78	79	80	81	81
12	119	120	121	123	124	125	126	79	79	79	80	81	82	82
13	121	122	123	124	126	127	128	80	80	80	81	82	83	83
14	123	123	125	126	127	129	129	81	81	81	82	83	84	84
15	124	125	126	127	129	130	131	82	82	82	83	84	85	85
16	125	126	127	128	130	131	132	82	82	83	84	85	85	86
17	125	126	127	129	130	131	132	82	83	83	84	85	85	86

Source: http://www.nhlbi.nih.gov/guidelines/hypertension/child_tbl.htm (accessed 7/24/04).

BODY MASS INDEX CONVERSION TABLE

Height in inches (cm)	BMI 25 kg/m^2	BMI 27 kg/m^2	BMI 30 kg/m^2
	Body weight in pounds (kg)		
58 (147.32)	119 (53.98)	129 (58.51)	143 (64.86)
59 (149.86)	124 (56.25)	133 (60.33)	148 (67.13)
60 (152.40)	128 (58.06)	138 (62.60)	153 (69.40)
61 (154.94)	132 (59.87)	143 (64.86)	158 (71.67)
62 (157.48)	136 (61.69)	147 (66.68)	164 (74.39)
63 (160.02)	141 (63.96)	152 (68.95)	169 (76.66)
64 (162.56)	145 (65.77)	157 (71.22)	174 (78.93)
65 (165.10)	150 (68.04)	162 (73.48)	180 (81.65)
66 (167.64)	155 (70.31)	167 (75.75)	186 (84.37)
67 (170.18)	159 (72.12)	172 (78.02)	191 (86.64)
68 (172.72)	164 (74.39)	177 (80.29)	197 (89.36)
69 (175.26)	169 (76.66)	182 (82.56)	203 (92.08)
70 (177.80)	174 (78.93)	188 (85.28)	207 (93.90)
71 (180.34)	179 (81.19)	193 (87.54)	215 (97.52)
72 (182.88)	184 (83.46)	199 (90.27)	221 (100.25)
73 (185.42)	189 (85.73)	204 (92.53)	227 (102.97)
74 (187.96)	194 (88.00)	210 (95.26)	233 (105.69)
75 (190.50)	200 (90.72)	216 (97.98)	240 (108.86)
76 (193.04)	205 (92.99)	221 (100.25)	246 (111.59)

Metric conversion formula = weight (kg)/height (m^2)
Example of BMI calculation:
A person who weighs 78.93 kilograms and is 177 centimeters tall has a BMI of 25:
weight (78.93 kg)/height (1.77 m^2) = 25

Non-metric conversion formula = [weight (pounds)/height (inches^2)] × 704.5
Example of BMI calculation:
A person who weighs 164 pounds and is 68 inches (or 5' 8") tall has a BMI of 25:
[weight (164 pounds)/height (68 inches^2)] × 704.5 = 25

Source: Adapted from NHLBI Obesity Guidelines in Adults, 1998.

ESTIMATE OF 10-YEAR CARDIAC RISK FOR MEN[a]

Age (y)	Points
20–34	−9
35–39	−4
40–44	0
45–49	3
50–54	6
55–59	8
60–64	10
65–69	11
70–74	12
75–79	13

Total Cholesterol	Points				
	Age 20–39	Age 40–49	Age 50–59	Age 60–69	Age 70–79
<160	0	0	0	0	0
160–199	4	3	2	1	0
200–239	7	5	3	1	0
240–279	9	6	4	2	1
≥ 280	11	8	5	3	1

	Points				
	Age 20–39	Age 40–49	Age 50–59	Age 60–69	Age 70–79
Nonsmoker	0	0	0	0	0
Smoker	8	5	3	1	1

HDL (mg/dL)	Points
≥ 60	−1
50–59	0
40–49	1
< 40	2

Systolic BP (mm Hg)	If Untreated	If Treated
< 120	0	0
120–129	0	1
130–139	1	2
140–159	1	2
≥ 160	2	3

Point Total	10-Year Risk %	Point Total	10-Year Risk %
< 0	< 1	9	5
0	1	10	6
1	1	11	8
2	1	12	10
3	1	13	12
4	1	14	16
5	2	15	20
6	2	16	25
7	3	≥ 17	≥ 30
8	4		

10-Year Risk _____ %

[a]Framingham point scores.

Source: U.S. Department of Health and Human Services, Public Health Service, National Institutes of Health, National Heart, Lung, and Blood Institute. NIH Publication No. 01-3305, May 2001.

ESTIMATE OF 10-YEAR CARDIAC RISK FOR WOMEN[a]

Age (y)	Points
20–34	−7
35–39	−3
40–44	0
45–49	3
50–54	6
55–59	8
60–64	10
65–69	12
70–74	14
75–79	16

Total Cholesterol	Points				
	Age 20–39	Age 40–49	Age 50–59	Age 60–69	Age 70–79
<160	0	0	0	0	0
160–199	4	3	2	1	1
200–239	8	6	4	2	1
240–279	11	8	5	3	2
≥ 280	13	10	7	4	2

	Points				
	Age 20–39	Age 40–49	Age 50–59	Age 60–69	Age 70–79
Nonsmoker	0	0	0	0	0
Smoker	9	7	4	2	1

HDL (mg/dL)	Points
≥ 60	−1
50–59	0
40–49	1
< 40	2

Systolic BP (mm Hg)	If Untreated	If Treated
< 120	0	0
120–129	1	3
130–139	2	4
140–159	3	5
≥ 160	4	6

Point Total	10-Year Risk %	Point Total	10-Year Risk %
< 9	< 1	17	5
9	1	18	6
10	1	19	8
11	1	20	11
12	1	21	14
13	2	22	17
14	2	23	22
15	3	24	27
16	4	≥ 25	≥ 30

10-Year Risk _____ %

[a]Framingham point scores.
Source: U.S. Department of Health and Human Services, Public Health Service, National Institutes of Health, National Heart, Lung, and Blood Institute. NIH Publication No. 01-3305, May 2001.

PROFESSIONAL SOCIETIES & GOVERNMENTAL AGENCIES		
Abbreviation	**Full Name**	**Internet Address**
AACE	American Association of Clinical Endocrinologists	http://www.aace.com
AAD	American Academy of Dermatology	http://www.aad.org
AAFP	American Academy of Family Physicians	http://www.aafp.org
AAHPM	American Academy of Hospice and Palliative Medicine	http://www.aahpm.org
AAO	American Academy of Ophthalmology	http://www.aao.org
AAOHNS	American Academy of Otolaryngology/Head & Neck Surgery	http://www.entnet.org
AAOS	American Academy of Orthopaedic Surgeons	http://www.aaos.org
AAP	American Academy of Pediatrics	http://www.aap.org
ACC	American College of Cardiology	http://www.acc.org
ACCP	American College of Chest Physicians	http://www.chestnet.org
ACIP	Advisory Committee on Immunization Practices	http://wonder.cdc.gov
ACOG	American College of Obstetricians and Gynecologists	http://www.acog.com
ACP	American College of Physicians	http://www.acponline.org
ACPM	American College of Preventive Medicine	http://www.acpm.org
ACR	American College of Radiology	http://www.acr.org
ACS	American Cancer Society	http://www.cancer.org
ACSM	American College of Sports Medicine	http://www.acsm.org
ADA	American Diabetes Association	http://www.diabetes.org
AGA	American Gastroenterological Association	http://www.gastro.org
AGS	American Geriatrics Society	http://www.americangeriatrics.org
AHA	American Heart Association	http://www.americanheart.org
AHRQ	Agency for Healthcare Research and Quality	http://www.ahrq.gov

PROFESSIONAL SOCIETIES & GOVERNMENTAL AGENCIES (CONTINUED)		
Abbreviation	**Full Name**	**Internet Address**
AMA	American Medical Association	http://www.ama-assn.org
ANA	American Nurses Association	http://www.nursingworld.org
AOA	American Optometric Association	http://www.aoanet.org
ASCRS	American Society of Colon and Rectal Surgeons	http://www.fascrs.org
ASCO	American Society of Clinical Oncology	http://www.asco.org
ASGE	American Society for Gastrointestinal Endoscopy	http://www.asge.org
ASHA	American Speech-Language-Hearing Association	http://www.asha.org
ATA	American Thyroid Association	http://www.thyroid.org
ATS	American Thoracic Society	http://www.thoracic.org
AUA	American Urological Association	http://auanet.org
CDC	Centers for Disease Control and Prevention	http://www.cdc.gov
CNS	Canadian Congress of Neurological Sciences	http://www.ccns.org
CTF	Canadian Task Force on Preventive Health Care	http://www.ctfphc.org
GAPS	Guidelines for Adolescent Preventive Services	http://www.ama-assn.org/ama/upload/mm/39/gapsmono.pdf
NAPNAP	National Association of Pediatric Nurse Practitioners	http://www.napnap.org
NCI	National Cancer Institute	http://cancer.gov/cancerinformation
NEI	National Eye Institute	http://www.nei.nih.gov
NGC	National Guidelines Clearinghouse	http://www.guidelines.gov
NHLBI	National Heart, Lung, and Blood Institute	http://www.nhlbi.nih.gov
NHPCO	National Hospice and Palliative Care Organization	http://www.nhpco.org

PROFESSIONAL SOCIETIES & GOVERNMENTAL AGENCIES (CONTINUED)		
Abbreviation	**Full Name**	**Internet Address**
NIDR	National Institute of Dental and Craniofacial Research	http://www.nidr.nih.gov
NIHCDC	National Institutes of Health Consensus Development Conference	http://www.consensus.nih.gov
NIP	National Immunization Program	http://www.cdc.gov/nip
NOF	National Osteoporosis Foundation	http://www.nof.org
NTSB	National Transportation Safety Board	http://www.ntsb.gov
SCF	Skin Cancer Foundation	http://www.skincancer.org
SGIM	Society for General Internal Medicine	http://www.sgim.org
SVU	Society for Vascular Ultrasound	http://www.svunet.org
USPSTF	United States Preventive Services Task Force	http://www.ahrq.gov/clinic/uspstfix.htm

REFERENCES

The Canadian Task Force on the Periodic Health Examination: The Canadian Guide to Clinical Preventive Health Care. Minister of Public Works and Government Services Canada, 1994. (Referred to as "CTF" in tables). Updated guidelines available at: http://www.ctfphc.org.

Elster AB (ed): American Medical Association. AMA Guidelines for Adolescent Preventive Services (GAPS): Recommendations and Rationale. Williams & Wilkins, 1994. (Referred to as "GAPS" in tables)

Bright Futures: Guidelines for Health Supervision of Infants, Children, and Adolescents. Bright Futures at Georgetown University. 2nd ed, rev. 2002. (http://www.brightfutures.org) (Referred to as "Bright Futures" in tables)

U.S. Preventive Services Task Force: Guide to Clinical Preventive Services, 2nd ed. Williams & Wilkins, 1996. (Referred to as "USPSTF" in tables) Updated guidelines now available at: http://www.ahcpr.gov/clinic/uspstfix.htm.

Geriatrics at Your Fingertips. Blackwell Publishing, 2003. Online version: http://www.geriatricsatyourfingertips.org/.

Index